# THE HABITS OF
# HEALTH

## How To Get The Body You Want And Feel Amazing

# THE HABITS OF

# HEALTH

*How To Get The Body You Want And Feel Amazing*

## Lo Allariz

www.loallariz.com

Published by Lo Allariz

www.loallariz.com



Cover design by Matthew Ocampo, Mary Juliette, and Shane Palor

Printed by CreateSpace

ISBN-13: 978-1720735366

# Dedication

You are the master of your destination, and this is my dedication to all those who reflect and identify with the belief that everything is possible when you change your bad habits to healthy habits and work as a whole towards feeling amazing.

# Acknowledgments

I focused on the habit of showing gratitude. I recognised and acknowledged you, the reader. If you did not read my book, I would not write it. So, once again thank you.

Once the book started to go from a concept in my head to a manuscript, there was a special person involved who deserves to be acknowledged and thanked—my coach, Harry Sardinas. Without his input, I could not have completed this book.

I am grateful to Lily Patrascu for coming up with the title of the book.

The next step was to edit and proofread, and I want to thank my editor, Luanne Thibault.

I would like to thank the greatest cover designers: Matthew Ocampo, Mary Juliette, and Shane Palor.

I would like to thank other authors about the topic of my book: Dr Jason Fung, Dr Robert Lustig, Dr Michael Mosley, Nina Teucholz, Gary Taubes, and Charles Duteigg.  Throughout my research, their points of view and expertise have helped to shape my book, and it was of great value.

And finally, I would like to thank my family: my mother, Rosario Santiago Villanueva; my sister, Lourdes Allariz Santiago; my cousin, Mari Carmen Mella Santiago; my nieces, Mirta Maria

Santiago and Anxela Fernandez Allariz; my nephew, Iago Fernandez Allariz; my godson, Jorge Sabucedo Mella; and my friends Esther Seninde and Irene McGregor. To the rest of my family, my other sister and brother, my aunties, uncles, cousins, my other nephews, nieces, friends and colleagues from work, thank you all for letting me know that you had nothing but great memories of me.  They also instilled exceptional values in me, which are a great help to me in my present and future life. Once again, thank you.

# Table of Contents

# Foreword

Lo Allariz is a good example of someone with a great vision and determination to inspire and help others live a healthy life. When I met Lo, I was astonished by how motivated, driven, and ambitious Lo was to make a difference in the world.

She has shown everyone, including myself, that anybody with a great vision can achieve anything they want—including turning their knowledge into a book, to inspire and motivate more and more people.

Have you ever had that feeling, that you wanted to save the world, but felt pretty helpless and, to a point, even disregarded the impact you could have made?

Well, Lo Allariz is making an impact in the world one step at a time, by helping people make minor changes in their health habits that lead to huge results in their life.

And you can do this too!

Lo Allariz is a Spanish nurse practitioner and a nutritional therapist member of the British Nutrition Foundation.

Her motto is: let your food be your medicine and your medicine be your food.

Have you ever wanted to lose weight, but you didn't know how to do it?

Or have you ever wanted to put on weight, but you simply had no clue where to start?

The key element missing is the right balance in your food.

Lo is showing all of us in this book that it can be very easy to start getting the body you want with some small changes in your habits.

Lo is driven by an amazing goal to help the poorest people living without clean drinking water and in unsanitary conditions. Her mission is to eradicate water and hygiene problems by coming together to create an infrastructure to save lives. She believes every person deserves the right to live in the very best way.

I am thrilled and delighted to have inspired Lo to write her book, and I am very proud of what she has achieved. If you are someone who wants to live a life full of energy, and live your life to the fullest, buy Lo Allariz' book and start creating the health habits that will enable you to thrive!

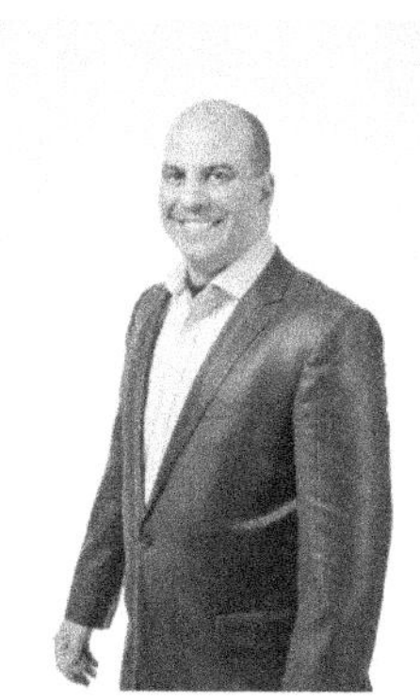

Harry Sardinas

Best-selling author of *Climbing Big Ben: How to Survive, Thrive and Succeed in London*.

www.HarrySardinas.com

www.SpeakersAreLeaders.com

www.BrandForSpeakers.com

# Preface

Hello, I am Ms Lo Allariz. I'm from Spain, and I currently live in England, where I did my training in nursing. I hold a Bachelor of Science in Critical Care degree, a postgraduate qualification in pathology and assessment of illnesses and injury conditions; and a Leadership and Management in Healthcare and Scope of Advanced Healthcare Practice certificate. I am a member of the Nursing Midwifery Council and the Royal College Council. I am currently working as a nurse practitioner, and I have worked in the field of nursing for over fifteen years. I have also worked as a volunteer nurse in different projects in Africa and South America.

I am also a nutritional therapist. I have been passionate about the importance of the food that we eat since I was a teenager. My philosophy is to make the food that you eat to be your best medicine and let your medicine be the food that you eat for a healthy and long life. The key is to eat a balanced diet and avoid junk/fast food/sugary drinks. I am also passionate about encouraging people to believe in themselves to be able to create better and healthier eating habits. I am a member of the British Nutrition Foundation, the Health Science Academy, and a subscriber to Harvard Medical School.

This book is written to help you to develop healthier habits and have that amazing life that you always wanted. I would like you to contribute how to implement proper practices, because I want you to create a healthier life for yourself and your loved ones. I want you to develop a life of purpose of trying to help you to lose your pounds and not your life. If you create something where you are contributing, you will feel good about it. My intention is not only to help you to face some of your regular problems but also to do it in a more automatic and healthy way. I hope to help you to establish some good habits that you need to implement to be happier and feel good about yourself.

What do you want from your life? And, what do you want for your loved ones?

Focus your conscious mind about what you want for yourself and those around you. One of the main aspects of being a human is the food that we eat. From our very first moment on this planet, the first thing we do is eat. We know how to feed ourselves as soon as we are born thanks to our excellent instinct for survival.

In our infancy, we had nourishing breastfeeding. But, as we grew up, we spoilt our appetite with junk food. This worries me, because to remain a healthy human, it is vital to eat proper food. People do not realise, but the way and how we feel depends very much on what we eat. When we eat junk food, it can make us feel drowsy and lethargic. On the other hand, when we eat fruits or vegetables, it can make us feel more energetic. What I am trying to say is that the food that we eat is the best medicine we need for a healthy and amazing life. Or, if we do not eat the proper foods, what we eat can poison us.

Think about you and your children and not eating the right food; it has consequences. Obesity has become a big problem in our society. Always remember that not all the foods in the supermarkets are good for you. Please, do not let society automate you and dictate what you eat. Be yourself by implementing amazing habits of knowledge and wisdom to improve your patterns of eating the proper food.

In the developing countries, people die because of a lack of water and food. In the developed nations, people die due to an excess of food intake and the co-morbidities that they carry with them.

Life is passing by. Sometimes I think that it appears close and other times it looks so far, so distant. And then I realise that life is not far or close from us, but within us, within our mind, spirit, intelligence, perception, and how to build our habits, and we can make the most of them. Life is too precious, and we need to grasp and enjoy it at every single moment. Our past has gone, and our future has yet to come, so we are left with the current time.

People need to be more aware of what they eat and the kind of food they consume, and they should know how damaging certain foods can be for themselves and their children, children that may still be developing their heart, liver, kidneys, or lungs. So, people need to know about the importance of having a proper and balanced diet with amazing habits to help them to achieve this. We live in a society of pleasure, and now everything seems to be allowed. But always remember this quote and the way you want to make a difference with you and your body:

Take care of your body.
It is the only place you have to live. —Jim Rohn

That quote had a real impact on me; I was a teenager at that time. That quote changed my life and my eating habits. At that moment, I knew I had to look after my body very seriously. Since then, I have eaten proper food, as I knew that if I didn't look after my body, nobody else would do it for me. That phrase by Jim Rohn had a real effect on me, and I was so astonished by its true content, that it will be with me for the rest of my life.

I have always been conscientious of looking after my body very well; since it is the unique thing that belongs to us in this world. My body deserves a lot of respect on my behalf; I feel it is a privilege to care for it in the best way possible and never take it for granted.

I've seen family members and friends destroy their bodies through alcohol, smoking, or overeating. And I've seen how they slowly ruined their lives and their desire to live.

Nowadays, more than ever, to be overweight and obese has become an epidemic. Even though I have never had problems with being overweight, I was affected closely by my family members, and, in particular, my mother who has always been overweight. I have also had friends and work colleagues that kept trying to lose weight. My family and friends kept trying different methods. One day they would decide on one diet; the next day they would try another one. They even tried to exercise more, and unfortunately, the list seemed to be endless. It broke up my heart to see them like that, because I could see their suffering.

So, as Mahatma Gandhi said, You must be the change you wish to see in the world.

With part of the profits from this book, I intend to donate part of the benefits to a charity organisation (Water Aid). They help the poor and needy in developing countries with drinking water and sanitation conditions. Thank you for your faithful support and help to improve their lifestyle. Your compassion enriches their lives in more ways than you'll ever know. Let's help them to start building good eating habits too!

# Chapter 1:
# How Do You Create New Habits

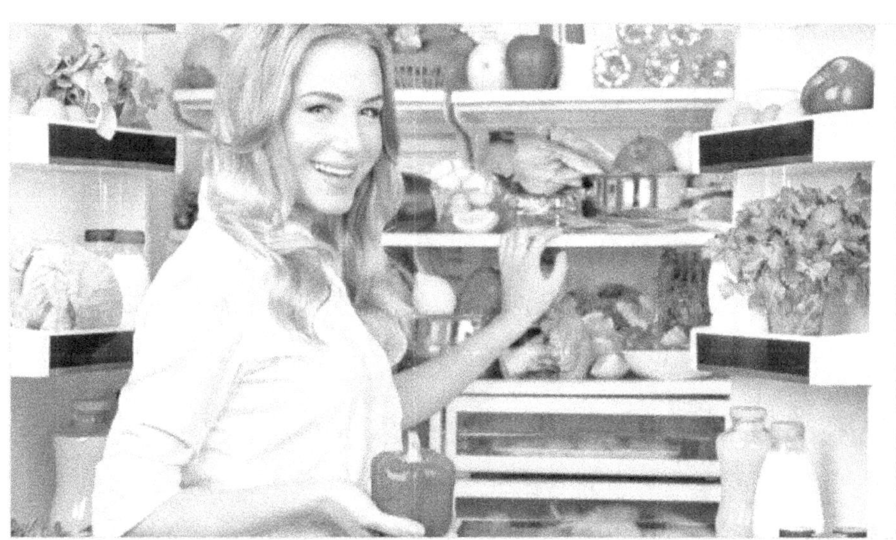

Start with new habits by putting
healthy foods in your refrigerator

# 1.1 - What is a habit?

To help us to understand better how our habits are formed, we will refer to different studies shown in this field. Researchers mention that all habits have the same circles and follow a typical pattern: a cue/reminder, routine, and reward habit circles. One thing to bear in mind is that there is a lot of science behind the process of habit formation.

As an example of how a habit works, let's see the steps that a habit follows in a typical phone call:

Step one is the cue/reminder. The simple fact the phone is ringing triggers a reminder, which is to reply to that phone call.

Step two is routine. The fact that we return to that phone call manifests a behaviour and, therefore, we demonstrate a habit to answer that phone call.

Step three is a reward. Once you answer that phone call, you finally find out who called, which is the manifestation of your curiosity of knowing who was behind that phone call and why she or he called you. This final step is called the reward.

To summarise this illustration, the reward, which is the end step of the habit cycle that we all have, is based on behaviour that tells your brain how to behave. So, to respond again to a phone call, you have to do the same thing all over again! Once we repeat these same steps, the way our brain works is that we stop thinking about it and our behaviour has turned into a habit.

Therefore, your behaviour becomes a habit that automatically does things without thinking, and here is where the key is to build up our new good habits.

The million-dollar question is: 'How can I stick to new and good habits and forget my old ones?'

This is the trick—we can use our present habit as a reminder to turn it into a new practice.

Many people think that to implement a new habit, you need self-control or you need to have a high dose of willpower.

But I disagree with these comments. The worst thing one can do to change and implement new habits is get motivated and then try to remember to take new steps. It is precisely the wrong way to go about it, because, sometimes you feel motivated and sometimes you don't, right? So, the way to go about it and create a new habit should not rely on motivation (something that changes). To create a new habit, one needs to be consistent. This is why the reminder—the trigger for your new behaviour—is such an essential element of building new habits. An important reminder makes it easier for you to start your practice by encoding your modern method in something that you already do, rather than relying on getting motivated.

Let me illustrate this to you with an example. Studies revealed that the practice of brain exercises can help you to reduce mental health diseases like Alzheimer's. We always want to avoid developing mental health problems. According to studies, a suitable method that could help us to postpone diseases like Alzheimer's is about doing brain exercises.

What are brain exercises? They are also known as neurobics for your mind. This term means tasks that activate the brain's biochemical pathway and brings new paths that can help to strengthen or preserve brain circuits.

A simple example for me to put some of the brain exercises in practice, would be to brush my teeth, *but* with my non-dominant hand, my left hand. I need to get into the habit of brushing my teeth with my other hand. As I am not used to brushing my teeth with my left hand, this will help my brain to intertwine new paths and help to form and strengthen new brain circuits. Doing these brain exercises helps with mental agility. And people with psychological agility tend to have lower rates of age-related mental decline.

Neurobics is a different new science of brain exercises. What these brain exercises do is that they use your five physical senses and also the emotional feeling that encourages you to shake up your everyday routine. These practical exercises do not require puzzles or paper and pens. It works by performing the task every day. The daily life routines, like eating or shopping or relaxing, can be done anywhere and at any time in offbeat. They are encouraged to help your brain to preserve, strengthen, and grow new brain cells.

The same thing happens with another practical neurobics exercise. Try this as an exercise. Close your eyes and use your other senses of touch, smell, and spatial memory to unlock and enter your home. The rationale behind this is that while doing this new routine, it becomes an exercise to your brain, as your underused nerve pathways and connections get activated. Consequently, the production of these connections helps your nerve cell receivers (dendrites) stay in better shape. This contributes to having a fit and flexible mind well prepared to face any mental challenge, whether it be playing chess or remembering a name.

With the way our senses work, smell, taste, touch, hearing, and vision each have their own sections in the brain. Our senses are very important in our daily life, and it is essential to use them. If you do not use them, you can create a mental traffic jam, and that may lead you to think, Oh no! I'm losing it! The neurobic program is a natural and straightforward way to encourage those mental toll booths to open, so your neuronal lanes remain in form, flexible, and ready for smooth traffic. Also, by practising these exercises, they help to keep your brain's pathways active, and that helps to create brain food known as neurotrophins (they belong to a kind of family of proteins, which regulate the development, maintenance, and function of neurons).

Thus, you can create and automate a new habit and have fun and exercise your brain at the same time. By enhancing the other senses and practising neurobic exercises, we take the brain out of its comfort zone. By changing our daily routine, we can improve our brain function. So, try something new! It doesn't have to be complicated; simple habit exercises can have great results and lead you to amazing cognitive functions.

Other neurobic exercises to maintain mental fitness and prevent memory loss are showering with your eyes closed, switching around your morning activities, turning familiar objects upside down, switching seats at the table, playing with spare change, or opening the car window.

Thus, we can develop habits without much effort or motivation. The key is that we need to automate them in our sub-consciousness like when we drive a car.

## 1.2 - What are the habits that destroy your life?

We all want to live a healthy, happy, and fulfilling life, yet so few of us achieve that.

We keep trying when a new year starts, and its respective New Year's resolution to change our habits. And yet we continue falling into all those patterns that destroy our lives like eating junk food, smoking, or a lack of exercise. But, why? Why is it so hard to stick to those new habits if they will help us to have a more fulfilling life?

Our brains function in different ways in our determination to change our habits. Whether we are motivated or not, we need to break a bad habit and replace it with a good habit. Whether or not we can change depends on the way we make those changes in the right or wrong way. Let me explain.

Stop smoking and start breathing fresh air.

Find a job that you enjoy rather than showing up to a job you hate every day.

Stop biting your nails, and remove any stress from your life.

Stop watching TV; start going to the gym.

We need to transform all these habits, to make us happier and more energised. Remember that all the habits that you have are a product of many small decisions that you made over time. Our brain has made every single decision throughout our lifetime, and the problems you are facing are the result of thousands of small choices over the course of years.

Habits are formed over the years, and those habits can be bad or good ones. Think about it—how happy or unhappy are you? How successful or unsuccessful are you?  How fit or not fit are you? All these conclusions are the result of your habits. When you do something repeatedly every day, they turn out to be your habits. What you do every day and what you think about usually determines the kind of person you are, your beliefs, and the personality you show.

The big mistake people make is that they set their sights on an overnight success or transformation, or they want to obtain a quick fix or achievement. They don't realise that they need to be focused more on their habits and routines, and that takes time. I want you to stick to your aims of a long-term reward by implementing and adhering to new good habits. The main thing is to keep getting better and better with your habits and keep learning how to master them.

I decided to learn more about how I could change and implement new habits. I discovered a helpful blend of academic research and real-world experiences that have allowed me to make progress in many areas of life, and this takes time. I wanted to reflect this manifestation of my development with you throughout this book.

## 1.3 - How do you build a new habit and avoid the old one?

Setting up a visible reminder and linking my new habit with a current behaviour made it much easier to switch to the correct habit, such as the brain exercises. There was no need to be motivated. There was no need to remember. They can be automated.

Of course, I'm not saying it's going to be easy. If you want to stick to the new behaviour that you want to transform in your life (like eating healthier or working out), the first step to consider is to put in practice a program that makes it easier for you to start. And for that reason, choosing the correct reminder for your new habit is the first step.

You need to choose to initiate your new behaviour, which is pretty much specific to each of you, according to your lifestyle and the new habit you are trying to create.

I discovered that a good reminder for my new habit is to write down two lists. In one list, I write the things I do routinely without fail. For instance, brush my teeth, have my breakfast, or sit down for dinner. Those actions can act as reminders for new health habits. For example, after I drink my natural orange juice in the morning, I implement a new behaviour, such as meditating for three minutes. I know it's a small habit, but this is the way to apply a pattern entirely, as those three minutes can expand to seven and then ten minutes without putting much effort throughout the next few weeks.

The second list that I write down is about the things that happen to me each day, for instance, watching a commercial on TV. These happenings can also act as triggers for my new habit. For instance, when a commercial comes on TV, I do four push-ups.

By writing down these two lists, you can see there is a wide range of things that you already do, and you already act on them every day. Those are the perfect reminders for new habits that can be automated.

For another example, let's say you want to feel happier. Showing gratefulness is one proven way to boost happiness. Putting the lists above into practice, you could select the prompt sit down for dinner and take it as a cue to say one thing that you are grateful for that day. When I meditate every morning, I always show my appreciation of life and the opportunity for another day to be in this universe. This little behaviour or attitude is the one that makes a difference that could blossom into more grateful outlooks on life in general.

I would like to share with you a quote by Babauta: Make your habit incredibly easy to start. Make it so easy you can't say no.

It is always a good reminder to start small if somebody wants to start a new habit, and they are willing to start a healthier life.

Now, choose a new habit you want to start and ask yourself, 'How can I make this new behaviour so easy to do that I can't say no?'

It is also a good idea to reward yourself when you're trying to create a new habit. Tell yourself phrases of encouragement. For instance, if I'm working towards a new self-development goal, then I'll often say to myself at the end of my reading session, that was an inspiring reading, or excellent job, or everything I hoped for.

It is also encouraging, for instance, if you tell yourself well done for every single thing you do when you start a new habit.  Give yourself some credit and enjoy each small success.

I must admit that habits appear to me as a revelation in relation to how habits dictate almost everything we do. I realised after reading books about habits that all we want to achieve in life, with regard to our personal growth and endeavours in life, depends on our ability to identify, reshape, and build our habits.

A quote from Aristotle said, 'We are what we repeatedly do. Excellence, then, is not an act, but a habit.'

Habits are a powerful weapon that we can use to our benefit. They can help us to achieve our goals. The more you understand how a habit works, the less importance you will assign to willpower—the willpower that is manifested by the ability to control our thoughts and the way in which we behave. Thus, it is much more efficient to automate willpower, which leads to habits. For instance, it is more efficient to focus on a habit of doing push-ups for five minutes at seven in the morning on a daily basis, than to set up a goal of losing six pounds over the next two months.

As part of this book, I would also like to introduce you to THE AMAZING SYSTEM.

THE AMAZING system stands for:

**A** = Avoid not being the master of your life

**M** = Mind-set and inner peace

**A** = Access to new habits

**Z** = Zap negativity

**I** = Innovation with ways of eating, superfoods, and exercise

**N** = No, when you have to say no

**G** = Generate value by sharing

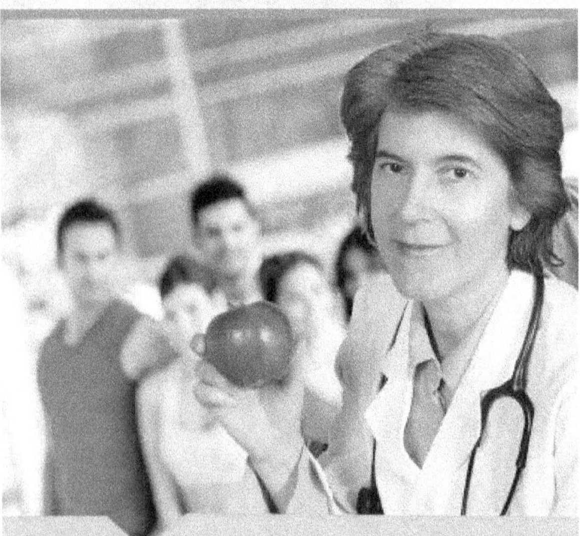

THE HABITS OF
HEALTH
AMAZING
- AVOID NOT BEING THE MASTER OF YOUR LIFE
- MINDSET AND INNER PEACE
- ACCESS TO NEW HABITS
- ZAP NEGATIVITY
- INNOVATION WITH WAYS OF EATING, SUPERFOODS AND EXERCISE
- NO, WHEN YOU HAVE TO SAY NO
- GENERATE VALUE BY SHARING
LO ALLARIZ
AUTHOR | HEALTH COACH | SPEAKER
email: hello@loallariz.com
www.loallariz.com

Thus, the A stands for: Avoid not being the master of your life. There are two ways of living your life. The first one is as a victim and the second one is as a master. You choose. While the former is about getting upset and angry at what life throws at you, and trying to change people and circumstances around you to make life easier, the latter is about taking whatever life throws at you and using it to change yourself, making yourself stronger and more adaptable, so life becomes easier and easier. Know that it will take time to have a transformational lifestyle. So, please do not be a victim, and keep persevering in making things happen towards creating good habits that will help you to create a better life for you and your loved ones.

The M stands for Mind-set and Inner Peace, which for me, was to transform my fixed mind-set to a growth mind-set. This transformation gave me the opportunity to easily automate my good habits to my sub-conscious mind, which then automatically made those habits as effortless as possible.

The A stands for Access to New Habits. To generate and achieve new habits, it is vital to have fun, have real conviction, and make them amazingly easy. So, make it accessible to you, to your comfort and your abilities.

The *Z* stands for Zap negativity or resistance. In all our journeys, we will face resistance and negativity, and to create new habits is not going to be different. But, and this is a BIG *but*, during moments like this is when you need to show who is in control, and don't let that your negativity or resistance control you.

The I stands for Innovation with Ways of Eating, Superfoods, and Exercise. Be the one to innovate yourself to create good habits. Don't let others influence you. Have the determination of being a new you with your new and amazing habits to become a better you.

The *N* stands for No. We need to say no to temptations, to people, and to things in life that are going to jeopardise our body, mind, and spirit.

The G stands for Generate value by Sharing with those you care about, by implementing and creating good habits for yourself. It can also be an inspiration for others around you, and, therefore, you can generate value for them, and all of you can have AMAZING results.

This system is a simple and straightforward system. It is based on the daily routine lifestyle that each of us has, and my purpose is to create habits and make them comfortable and accessible to you as an individual. I would also like to emphasise that it is not only about doing things but also about making things better for our own good.

I would like to share with you something about myself and how I had to face new habits that I wanted to implement to make things better in my life. And, yes, in all those new habits that I was involved in, there were times when I felt like a victim and, the more I thought about how hard it was to implement a new/good habit, the more victimized I felt. Then, I decided to stop being a victim, mainly because it wasn't working. One of the tools that helped me to stop being a victim was to realise that I want to be the master of my life rather than the victim.

It is your mind-set that has a great potential to affect your success or failure in life and help you to have an inner peace. Your mind-set shapes the way you perceive the world. Your mind is divided into a fixed or growth mind-set. I realised that I had a fixed mind-set, and I was determined to change my fixed mind-set to a growth mind-set. One of the strategies that I used was the implementation of new habits. Your habits make you who you are, because you can take control, and you are able to choose which behaviours, actions, and thoughts will become habits. Thus, I made sure that I had one habit well established before I started a new one, and then I moved forward and took that one habit further in life to a new and amazing life.

I have a snapshot in my daily routine, and then I decide what is the easiest and most accessible way to implement any new healthy habit. You can do that too.

With regard to zapping negativity, what really helped me was to put into practice and set up the habit of Mindfulness. I zapped the negativity or resistance and transformed it into acceptance. I changed it to a great deal of positivity and possibility in every single habit that I wanted to introduce in my life. The habit of Mindfulness helped me to zap those negative thoughts.

Like with everything in life, I also had to Innovate about how to sharpen my mind with ways of eating, superfoods, and exercise. I can say that, for instance, by putting in practice some previous exercises and practices, I managed to Automate them into my subconscious more and more. So, in this case, I implemented habits effortlessly and with a great deal of simplicity, and this could work on any single habit.

During this process, it was hard to say No. It was challenging, and, many times, I was beaten by all the distractions and temptations of the old, bad habits. But then, I wanted to get over it and to determine what I wanted to do with my life. Did I want to stick to my old habits and let them continue to ruin my life? Or, did I want to move forward and make myself a better person?

The skill that I most appreciated during my transformation of changing habits was that I could Generate value by sharing my experiences with others and how I could help and encourage others to pursue the body they wanted to feel AMAZING.

# Chapter 2: How to Overcome Hunger and Anxiety

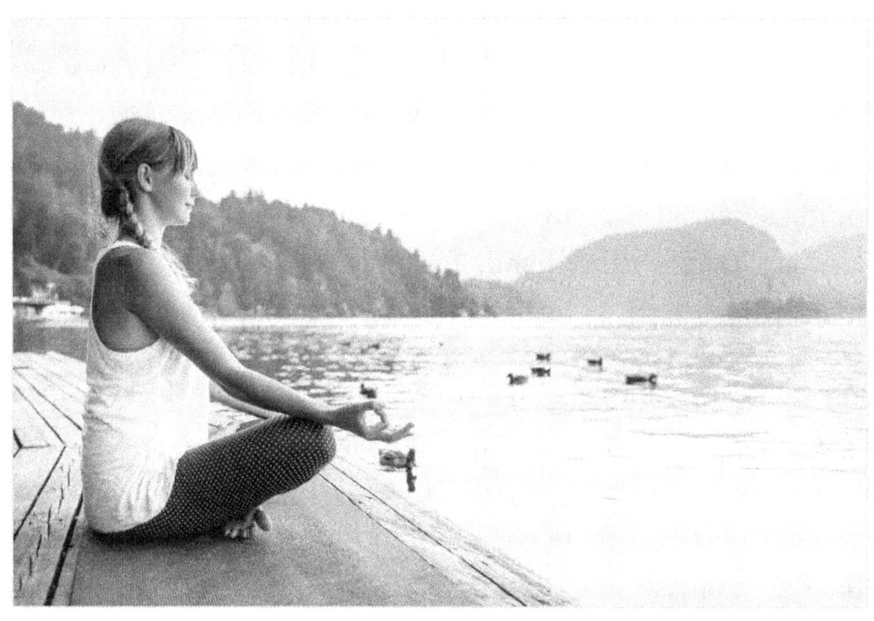

Meditation helps you to reduce your anxiety

## 2.1 - How can we control hunger?

Feeling hungry all the time can be harmful to your waistline. Do you know that it is not the calories that you intake that satiate your hunger? It is nutrients such as protein, healthy fats, and fibre that satiate your hunger.

Fibre is a great benefit for a ravenous appetite, it promotes gut health, and it also contributes to reducing the risk of developing many chronic diseases. Furthermore, it helps with the prevention of haemorrhoids, constipation, diverticulosis, and it has some properties that lower the risk of developing some cancers, such as bowel and breast cancer. Moreover, high-fibre foods have a lower glycaemic index value, an important element in managing type 2 diabetes.

Foods high in fibre are fresh fruits, legumes, vegetables, and nuts. High fibre foods tend to take a while to make it through your digestive tract. Soluble fibres contained in avocados, sweet potatoes, and tofu absorb water, forming a gel that slows digestion. On the other hand, insoluble fibres like those found in lentils, wheat bran, or beans are bulky and fill your belly.

Unfortunately, simple, refined carbohydrates are lacking in all three.  So, for example, many 100-calories snacks will fill your body with fast, cheap calories, but, no matter how much you eat, your body will go in search of more food. The outcome is a hungrier, sluggish you. Refined carbohydrates such as cookies, pancakes, pies, and pastries are rapidly absorbed into the bloodstream, causing risky spikes in blood sugar and insulin levels. The most common chronic diseases of Western civilization, like diabetes and obesity, have been tied to these types of deliciously addictive carbohydrates. Therefore, it is wise to keep them to a minimum.

Thus, eat real food and avoid the refined, processed, nutrient-depleted stuff. The more nutritious your food intake is, and the fewer empty calories you consume, the happier and more amazing your body will be. And this leads to a healthier metabolism with less intense hunger signals.

When we are born, all of us have an innate sense of hunger. Hunger is identified as a painful sensation of weakness produced by the lack of food. Some individuals may feel irritable, shaky, disoriented, lethargic, or lightheaded if they don't have their usual meals at specific times. However, the majority of people can tolerate it very well without eating and skip one, two, or even three meals of the day. As we will see in another chapter of this book, fasting is good for you.

Let me ask you something. Have you ever experienced a lunchtime when you thought that you were hungry but you became absorbed in a project or a book and several hours passed before you thought about food again? The definition of real hunger cannot wait a few hours. It demands to be fed. When you feel hungry in the afternoon, it is more related to a time-of-day stimulus rather than being hungry. If you occupy your mind with some other activity, the urge to eat usually passes within a few minutes. Therefore, bear in mind that there exists a big difference between your hunger urge and your real need for food.  And, of course, don't associate your emotional status with your food status. Please don't eat when you feel emotionally or physically uncomfortable; go for a walk or call one of your loved ones instead.

There are three different forms of hunger: mechanical, aesthetic, and chemical.

Mechanical hunger is the feeling of an empty stomach. This is the hunger that, if ignored for long enough, will go away altogether. Or, it will get uncomfortable and lead you to the desperation of chemical hunger.

Aesthetic hunger is the longing for food, but it is more than just needing the taste and physical feel of food. It is also eating for emotional reasons (comfort, nostalgia, grief, or celebration).

In ethnic foods, surveys revealed that the main reason people choose food is that of how it tastes. The need for enjoyment encourages people to look out for more flavours and it turns out to be a more nutritional variety, which is an essential component of nutritional excellence.

Chemical hunger is the type of hunger that goes beyond the garden-variety grumbly stomach. It is the sense that something is missing. I usually have this feeling when I have skipped two or three meals or not eaten enough of the vegetables or fruits I need for several meals or several days. When chemical hunger occurs, some people can feel weak or lightheaded. These are signals transmitted not only by the stomach but from your blood, your glycogen stores, and sometimes depleted vitamins and mineral stores.

When the chemical hunger is fulfilled, you will feel satisfied.

You will learn what you need to do to satisfy them. You will notice which foods give you an emotional lift, fulfil a flavour craving, and which foods and amounts give you the sense of fullness you like to have in your stomach.

Why do we ever stop eating?

Hunger is the interaction of different biochemical processes. Satiety in our body is influenced by the nutritional and metabolic state. It is related to our biochemical response to the absorption of nutrients and our access to stored nutrients.

Hunger helps to keep us alive, and not to make us fat. Hunger interaction is made of four principal biochemical and neurological motivations: likes, wants, satiation, and satiety.

In general terms, the meaning of satisfying hunger, satiation, and satiety are used interchangeably. However, they all have different aspects. Satiation is about the end of desire to eat after a meal. The responsibility for this effect are hormones and stretch receptors in the stomach. Thus, satiation signals the brain the meal is over. On the other hand, satiety is a physical sensation of fullness that allows you to stop eating for a while.

Satiation: it is a fact of our sensory and cognitive experience of eating.

The hedonic impact is the action and the pleasure and likes of ingesting food. Thus, *palatability* is the diabolic impact of food.

Incentive salience (wants) is a product of the other three motivations. It carries us to obtain something we like.

The other two elements that interact with hunger are *availability* and *willpower*.

For example, one might want roasted chicken much more than leftovers, but we eat the leftovers, because they are what is available to us. If I really want a roasted chicken, that is a trip to a store or a trip to a restaurant.

It is important to emphasise that *likes* and *wants* are not only in relation to the food we eat but also any other experiences we like that have a hedonic impact that is capable of producing a want for more incentive salience. The reward that we obtain when we eat is mixed together with the hedonic impact and incentive salience.

Our body is composed of cells and organs full of taste and nutrient receptors that sense the external and internal environment. Food intake is principally determined by its ability to produce satiation and satiety, not its hedonic impact.

Then we know that it is not our fault. We know that we are weak and foolish and cannot be trusted to make our own decisions. The responsibility lies with those corporations who have been making food that tastes too darned good, and we just cannot resist it.

But then, we realise that, yes, we are all part of this food industry, and, as consumers, we must stand for what will help us to have better health, not only for us but also for our loved ones.

An experiment was conducted where teenagers (lean and obese) had lunch at a mall. They could have pretty much whatever they liked, and the slim teenagers took practically the same amount as the obese teenagers. The primary outcome of this experiment found that both teenaged groups wanted the same amount of food. The difference was that the lean teenager's team compensated for that over the rest of the day. On the other hand, the obese kids did not. Therefore, this gives a strong suggestion that obesity is primarily a failure of satiety.

Our body not only has taste receptors situated in our tongues, but they are also located throughout our bodies. The pancreas releases insulin hormones. The intestines release satiety hormones like VIP (vasoactive intestinal peptide) or NPY (neuropeptide y). Other studies revealed that one could inject sugar into a rat and get the food reward effect, even though the rat never tasted the sugar. Thus, satiety is rewarding in itself. Therefore, by eating food that does not give satiety, you are chasing a reward that never comes. Does this sound familiar?

## How can we control hunger and anxiety?

There is a better and healthier way to feed your body and manage your hunger accordingly. It has worked for me and many others, and it can definitely work for you too. It involves getting back to eating real food—balanced meals and snacks—and limiting yourself to highly refined carbohydrates and eating good fat.

I am convinced that when you feed your body correctly, it has a chance to get back into balance with its hormones and metabolism. Once your body is in balance within itself—and I'm not talking only physically but mentally and spiritually—then your body works better and correctly, and the weight can melt away.

Research showed that leptin and ghrelin hormones are two compound chemicals that shape our appetite and hunger signals.

Leptin is made by adipose tissue and is secreted into the circulatory system, where it travels to the hypothalamus, whose main function is to link the nervous system to the endocrine system hormones/glands group). It is the leptin signals that send to the hypothalamus that we have enough fat, so we can stop eating or eat less. On the other hand, the ghrelin hormone is a short-term regulator of our body weight. Your stomach produces ghrelin when it is empty. And, just like leptin, ghrelin goes into the bloodstream, crosses the blood/brain barrier, and ends up at your hypothalamus, where it tells you that you are hungry.

Studies found that hunger can have an effect on memory for food-related stimuli where the orbitofrontal cortex is involved explicitly in food-related stimuli in a hunger state. Our food selection included biological factors of hunger, taste, and appetite; likewise to income and cost. Moreover, other factors that influence food choice are social and psychological elements of emotion, stress, and mood. Some Individuals find it hard to stop eating a particular food even though they are not hungry. This repetitive habit of eating comfort foods—with high fats, carbohydrates, and sugars—leads to obesity and that can develop into morbidity diseases, such as heart problems or diabetes.

## 2.2 - What is anxiety and how can we control it?

Anxiety is defined as an uneasy feeling, such as fear or worry. Unfortunately, more and more people suffer from feeling anxious. It becomes like an associate in our daily lives, so we try to cope with it the best way possible. Now the dilemma is how we deal with anxiety and whether it controls us or we manage it.

Anxiety can be an effect of being hungry, which, at the same time, can make you feel anxious. During our state of hunger and hypoglycaemia (low blood sugar) primitive signals have been known to set off the stress response in an individual.

Studies have found that stress can shut down your appetite in the short term, as it pumps out the hormone epinephrine (adrenaline). This hormone is responsible for the body's fight-or-flight response and puts eating on hold. However, if stress persists, it leads to a different effect, as the adrenal glands release a different hormone, known as cortisol, which will have an impact on your hunger hormones and will also pull lipids from your bloodstream to store them in your fat cells.

I genuinely believe that one's nutritional aspect of his/her life is crucial to achieving better anxiety health through diet. Studies have found that many dietary considerations can help relieve anxiety. For instance, have a balanced diet, make sure you are drinking enough water to stay hydrated, and avoid or limit alcohol and caffeine. In some foods, we find that complex carbohydrates are metabolized more slowly, and thus help to keep a more even blood sugar level, which creates a calmer feeling.

Thus, complex carbohydrates (brown rice, rye, oatmeal, or corn) are considered a better healthier option than having plenty of simple carbohydrates found in processed foods (white bread, sugary drinks, or table sugar).

More studies have revealed that the gut-brain axis is also essential as a significant amount (approximately 95%) of serotonin receptors are found in the lining of the gut. Your body produces serotonin chemicals that act on the nervous system, and it is related to feelings of well-being.

Studies have shown that foods rich in zinc—like liver, beef, or egg yolks—have been associated with lowering anxiety. Likewise, the same effect can happen if you eat foods that contain omega-3 fatty acids like fish.

Other foods considered to be anti-anxiety are beans, berries, vegetables, and nuts. And, two of the spices that contain antioxidants and anti-anxiety properties are ginger and turmeric.

Research revealed that the asparagus extract has terrific properties of anti-anxiety too. Consequently, the use of an asparagus extract was introduced as a natural functional food and beverage ingredient in the food industry.

The primary factor of the above foods—also known as feel good foods—is that they release neurotransmitters such as serotonin and dopamine. Serotonin is known as a compound chemical that it is found everywhere in our body, even in our gut. Thus, serotonin has different functions in our body, apart from making us feel relaxed, like dopamine does. Serotonin also helps us to regulate our memory, our body temperature, our sleeping patterns, and our appetite. The primary function of these neurotransmitters is to balance brain chemicals, thus reducing the number and severity of anxiety attacks. They are a safe and comfortable first step in managing anxiety. More and more, it is believed that the treatment options associated with diet help to maintain anxiety.

Dealing with anxiety can be a challenge and often requires making lifestyle changes. There aren't any diet changes that can cure anxiety, but watching what you eat may help you to reduce those stress levels.

While nutritional psychiatry is not a replacement for other psychological treatments, I indeed believe that the relationship between food, mood, and anxiety is getting more and more attention over the last few years.

About the soul-sucking feeling of anxiety, there is an elementary concept to be aware of:  if you want to fix a problem in your brain, you need to understand your brain.

Let's get started and make those habit changes in your life to get your anxiety under control.

I think the best habit one can apply to oneself is to change our mind-set. We are pretty much in this mood of pessimism, guilt, anxiety, and low self-esteem. Unfortunately, all these concepts are too familiar these days. Sadly, people find it far too easy to let these negative emotions get to them, keeping them down, feeling depressed and lonely. Now it's about time to get rid of all them; don't you think so?

## 2.3 - How do we create new and useful habits to stop hunger and anxiety?

A good tip to help you to reduce your hunger and feelings of depression is to drink a big glass of water and then wait approximately ten or fifteen minutes. After that time, your hunger should disappear.

Furthermore, water intake is an excellent habit of helping you to stop those hunger cravings and also to lose weight. A study found that participants who drank two 8-ounce glasses of water before breakfast, lunch, and dinner consumed, on average, 75 to 90 fewer calories at each meal. Thus, at the end of the twelve-week study, those participants lost about three kilos more than the participants in the control group, and it was only because they didn't feel as hungry, because of water's filling effect.

Eating too quickly is not a good idea either. You should try to implement a new habit of eating slowly. This is why: hunger hormones take between 20 to 30 minutes to get to your brain. So, if you eat too fast (in under 10 minutes), you will most likely eat more than you would have if you ate more slowly.

For many of us, hunger can be a real challenge. Each person needs to find his/her recipe for dealing with it.

Stress is the reason you can't lose weight. If one has a persistent fear, the adrenal glands release a hormone called cortisol. The main cortisol function is to trigger your hunger hormones, and it will also pull lipids from your bloodstream to store them in your fat cells. One method that helped me to manage stress is mindfulness or yoga. These two can be excellent strategies to help you to reduce your stress levels and introduce them as new habits too in your daily routine.

Another good habit is to stop eating when you are no longer hungry, and not when you feel full, or when nothing is remaining on your plate. As a good reminder, think about your clothes getting looser, and you'll start to enjoy leaving food on your plate or put smaller portions on your plate.

Always remember that a volume of non-nutritious food merely stuffs and bloats, but does not satisfy real hunger. On the other hand, variety and texture, along with nutritional food, satiate hunger.

For those folks re-learning good eating habits, it may take time, but stick with them; they work, and they are worthy. Be mindful of being patient with yourself. In the beginning, the results may get worse, physically or psychologically, before things improve, but it will get better, and it is excellent when it does.

I got into the habit of fasting once or twice a week. When I do fast, mechanical hunger is normal for me at intervals, and it is a beautiful feeling. I sometimes allow myself to feel it for a little while, to remind myself that it is fine and healthy and needs to be there.

I get to feel what normal hunger is and eat to fill my stomach.

Hunger is a fantastic mechanism, and I love that I finally got to experience it. This contributes to helping me to overcome the kind of feeling that my body is dying because my lunch is twenty minutes overdue. Eating is so much more straightforward and primal and far less anxiety-ridden. I love it.

You can diminish hunger signals if you ignore them or don't consistently respect them.

In our society, being hungry means merely a nagging grumble while we wait for dinner. However, for many children (right in your town), it says something much scarier, like not knowing when your next meal will come.

Let's be bland about this and say that this is something that is entirely within our control.

As we mentioned earlier on, it is essential to keep up a good diet where there is an increase of serotonin in a variety of foods, such as salmon, pineapples, cheese, nuts, eggs, or turkey. This healthy food will bring your brain chemistry back into balance. Thus, this can help you to stop feeling anxious, and you can start feeling amazing in both your body and your mind.

In general, an excellent habit to implement is to always keep up with a healthy diet, as it will help us to get in shape and limit unnecessary physical stress on our body.

A perfect refresher is that we need to remind ourselves again and again about how unsatisfied and hungry we feel after eating those fast-digesting carbohydrates, such as bread with refined flours and candies with added sugars. This kind of food is known as high glycaemic foods. To have better control of your appetite or satiety, you will need to have low glycaemic index foods. Also called low GI foods, they have the ability to increase the levels of a hormone that suppresses your appetite, making you feel full. During a study, researchers revealed that participants who ate a low glycaemic breakfast (such as eggs with spinach, or bran cereal, or yoghurt, or peanut butter) had an increased level of this hunger-fighting hormone than those who had high glycaemic foods (commercial bowls of cereal, sugar, flour, or bread).

Exercise is a good habit for our body; it's just the way we were made. This means that we were born to be mobile, and we should be mobile until the end of our days. When we are not active, our muscles get stiffer, and we become slow and lethargic. So, exercise keeps us healthy and, not only that, it helps to prevent hunger. When you work out, your body releases hormones that affect your appetite. Trained athletes often have lower appetites. Thus, when you exercise, blood moves away from your digestive tract and towards your muscles, preventing your belly from immediately signalling your brain that it is hungry.

Let me introduce my friend Ismael. Ismael has always had a struggle with his weight. He tried very hard to lose weight. He has been working different regimens and diets, and sometimes he lost weight and sometimes he put on. So, he was quite frustrated and stressed with himself. His frustration carried on throughout the years.

Now, more than ever he decided to be more motivated than ever to lose weight. He chose to be a good role model. He works in the social media field, and he wanted to change his image, in particular, get rid of those extra pounds.  I encouraged him to change his habits. He needed to get into the habit of reducing his soda/fizzy drinks, his sugary snacks, and his desserts and go for fresh and natural foods instead.

I truly believe that we do not need to follow any particular diet and just be sensible with what we eat. Ismael feels better now that he lost some weight with the implementation of a simple habit and without a great effort. Stick with the habit of eating fresh food, and avoid foods that do not give you any nutrients, like those soda or fizzy drinks. This helped him to reach his ideal weight and made him realise that, by investing a little effort, he could get amazing results that would lead to a healthier lifestyle.

# Chapter 3:
# Childhood Obesity

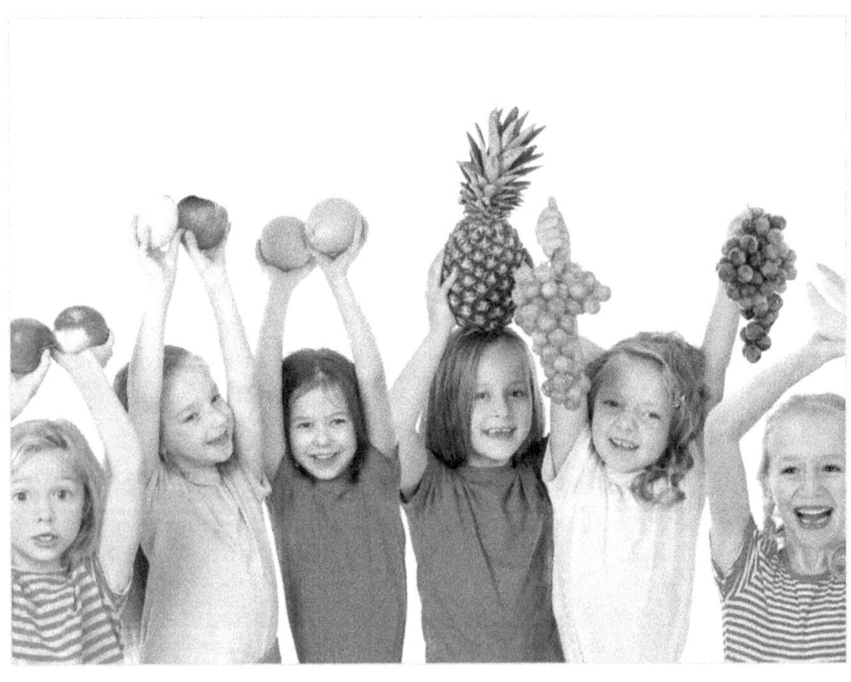

Start implementing healthy eating habits with your children

# 3:1 - What is obesity in children? and what is happening to our society that children are getting fat at a younger and younger age?

Obesity in children is when a child is grossly overweight or has a lot of fat.

The usual indicator if a child is overweight or obese is the BMI (Body Mass Index) percentiles. This means that the doctor compares a child's weight to others of the same age and sex. Thus, the BMI is the calculation of dividing an individual's weight in kilograms by the height in meters squared. A BMI percentile of 85% or less is a good weight. The percentages between 85% and 94% percentile are overweight, and above 95%, the child is considered obese.

Obesity in children has become an international epidemic. It has been revealed that there are around 124 million obese children.

Studies done worldwide revealed the increase in obesity over the last four decades went from 0.7% to 5.6%. And, if it continues on like this, child and teen obesity may even exceed severely overweight by 2022.

In England, one in five children are overweight or obese in reception school, and one in three children are overweight or obese in secondary school. Also, children in deprived areas have a higher tendency to be fat, and the gap has risen. Worldwide, the United Kingdom ranks sixth with childhood obesity at 27 %, and the USA ranks first with 38% of their children being severely overweight.

One of the reasons babies are fatter is because more expectant mothers are obese and the babies are born above a healthy weight range, and they develop childhood obesity, independent of any genetic or environmental factors. Children who are obese are more likely to be obese in adulthood. Subsequently, he/she will have more chances of having overweight or obese children later in life. Thus, other risk factors for gaining weight are poor diet due to a large amount of sugar ingesting and the decrease of exercise in general.

Moreover, researchers found that obesity is hormonal rather than a caloric imbalance. Insulin is the main hormonal component of weight gain. Insulin causes our newborn / infant / child / adult to put on weight and that leads to obesity.

For instance, where would an infant get high insulin? From his/her mother, as both of them share the same bloodstream. Thus, any insulin hormonal imbalance is directly transmitted through the placenta. We marinate our children in insulin beginning in the womb. Mothers with gestational diabetes mellitus tend to have three times more risk of suffering from a metabolic syndrome, which is a medical term for a combination of high blood pressure, diabetes, and obesity in later life.

In our environment, some factors contribute to obesity, such as the sale of supersized sugary drinks, refined, processed foods, and sugary snacking all the time, rather than increasing the consumption of vegetables and fruits. And this is the same kind of advice that you would get from your grandmother over fifty years ago, about losing weight: reduce sugars and starches. Cutting down on your snacking will help you to prevent high insulin levels, the key and central problem of obesity.

Also, research revealed that the intake of added sugars equably increased from 1977 along with obesity, leaving the undeniable truth remaining that sugar causes weight gain with hardly any nutritional values. The worst offender by far is the sugar-sweetened drink—soft drinks, sodas, juices, and sweetened teas. Soda is a $75 billion business. All these sugary drinks contribute to approximately 22% of the sugar found in the American diet.

Companies producing these sugar-sweetened drinks are now facing strong political opposition to outlaw oversized beverages. The beverage companies spent decades convincing people to drinking more soda or sweetened beverages. They became very successful, but at what cost? As obesity grew, these companies came under pressure from all sides, and, in particular, in America and Europe.

They then decided to sell their products to other markets in Asia to make up for lost profits from the Western countries. The consumption of sugar in Asian countries rises at almost 5% per year. The percentage of the population with diabetes type 2 in China was approximately 4% in 2000. Now, with the rise in sugar consumption, in 2013 approximately 11.6% of the Chinese adults were diagnosed with type 2 diabetes; this is around 22 million Chinese people, which is close to the entire population of Australia. China has eclipsed the rate of the long-time champion, the USA. Once again, researchers found that sugar more than other carbohydrate seems to be quite fattening and may lead to type 2 diabetes.

Why is sugar so fattening? Sugar is considered as empty calories, because it contains few nutrients, and it is fattening due to its nature as highly refined carbohydrates. It imbalances the insulin production, which leads to weight gain, like most refined carbohydrates, such as potatoes or rice. Moreover, sugar is a very palatable and rewarding food, and this may lead to overconsumption and obesity.

Studies showed obesity rose from 15% in 1993 to 27% in 2015.

The percentages of an increase in child obesity have skyrocketed recently. Statistics in the U.S. show that children between 6 and 11 years old, increased from 7% to 15.3%. Children between 12 to 15 years old rose even higher, up to 15.5% from 5% a few years ago. Moreover, studies have revealed the existing correlation between obesity and the rise in children with high blood pressure and type 2 diabetes.

Fast food meals contain a variety of unhealthy ingredients, including high fructose corn syrup. It can also be found in condiments like ketchup, soda, fries, salad dressings, mustard, and some bread products or desserts. The studies revealed that fructose corn syrup is an artificial sweetener, and it has been related to liver scarring, type 2 diabetes, and obesity.

A children's food campaign survey found that some baby food products may have just as much, if not more, saturated fats and sugar as junk food.

Furthermore, cheap table salt is also found in very large amounts in fast food, and this may lead to health problems and water retention.

Consequently, children are more prone to have high blood pressure, a fatty liver, type 2 diabetes, and sleep apnea, and the numbers are increasing. This increase is even more shocking when nutritionists and health care professionals take into consideration that it is mostly preventable.

So, that is why I am so passionate about what children need to eat. The best way to manage these health conditions is prevention in the first place. My motto, as Hippocrates, who is the father of medicine, quoted: let your food be your medicine and your medicine be your food.

Mind-set! The mind-set that our society has benefits the food industries, not the public. Parents provide their children with food, such as crisps, cookies, ice creams, or sugary drinks, and all these food products are detrimental to their health. But this is all about food marketing, marketing that bombards us on television, and social media on a regular basis. These types of foods can harm the little body of our children.

A child's body is still in the process of growing and developing. Their stomach, kidneys, and even their heart are not fully developed. Their bodies work much harder than adult bodies trying to get rid of so much salt and sugar that the junk food products contain. It is my aim to provide this information and defend those vulnerable children so they can eat healthier and more nutritious foods on a daily basis. Unfortunately, some parents are not fully aware of what harm junk food can do to their children's organs. They think that because this kind of food is in the market it is good enough to eat, and they don't  realise the serious consequences that they can bring their own children.

Nutritionists and physicians have shown that children are being diagnosed with high cholesterol and high blood pressure, and obese children have a double risk of developing hypertension, a fatty liver (a precursor to cirrhosis), obstructive sleep apnoea, or type 2 diabetes.

A recent study has also shown that back in 1990 the percentage of children with diabetes was less than 4%. Nowadays, the American Diabetes Association indicated that approximately 8-45% of children with newly diagnosed cases have nonimmune-mediated diabetes. This is terrifying as hardly twenty-five years have passed and the increase is so severe. This increase is even more shocking when health professionals consider that it is mostly preventable.

That is why I am so passionate about what children need to eat from the beginning of their lives. The foundation of a healthy mind-set and a way of eating proper food is vital to our children. Thus, the way we eat as adults, influences our children for the rest of their lives.

I am a health practitioner, and I treat many children with minor injuries or illness, and it breaks my heart to see children eating a bag of crisps or biscuits while I assess them. I can see they are a bit malnourished or overweight, and this is because they are not eating the proper food.  Parents could provide their children with better and healthier food, but they give junk food to their children. Parents are continuously bombarded by ads from food industries telling them to eat delicious and cheap food, but it is food with zero nutritional value. These food industries only care about their profit. So, we are helping them to get richer, while we get poorer and sicker.

In America's youth, the most significant threat is not cancer or opioid addiction but diabetes. A national Study showed that the number of children diagnosed with type 2—so-called adult diabetes—had increased considerably within a percentage of five percent every year between 2002 and 2012.

The Centers for Disease Control and Prevention reckon that one in three Americans will have diabetes by 2050. The condition can lead to other devastating health problems. For instance, half of all individuals who have diabetes will die from heart disease. Also, diabetes causes nearly half of all cases of kidney failure.

Furthermore, diabetic patients have a higher tendency of suffering from depression—more than twice that of non-diabetic people.

There is a saying, The best way to manage the disease is to prevent it in the first place. One useful tool against the condition is education. Some YMCAs (Young Men's Christian Associations) have implemented a program that trains overweight children how to eat healthier foods. After a year of the program, the results were terrific. The contestants managed to decrease their body-mass indexes, and they had a better regulation of their blood sugar levels.

The obesity epidemic is affecting younger and younger children, even in the zero-to-six-month-old age range. There are different hypotheses as to the cause of obesity. One hypothesis is the conventional calorie-based diet. Obesity is seen as an energy-balance problem. Then there's the *eating less and move more* theory. But, a six-month-old eats on demand, and it is usually breastfed. So, it is impossible that they could overeat. And, as a child at this age doesn't walk, it is impossible for them to exercise. So, what is happening? And how can newborn obesity be explained.

Now, more and more health professionals are wondering if obesity is more of a hormonal imbalance than a calorie imbalance and how the reduction of calories and exercising more method throughout these past decades has not shown much difference in losing weight.

Insulin is the main hormonal vehicle for weight gain. Insulin can cause obesity in a newborn, and, in general, can cause obesity in children and adults. I have a question: where would an infant get high insulin levels? It has to be from his/her mother. The foetus and the mother share the same blood supply. So, any hormonal imbalance, like high insulin levels, is transmitted to the foetus via the placenta.

The origins of childhood obesity are due to the high levels of insulin. The children of mothers who suffered gestational diabetes mellitus are more prone to develop obesity and diabetes in later life.

Scientific research also found that there is a higher risk for children born to mothers who were overweight or obese prior to pregnancy, and they are more prone to have autism, cognitive developmental delays, or deficit disorders.

More and more researchers focus on the reduction of snacks and sugar, rather than reducing fat and calories. Cutting down sugars and starches will attack the worst offenders of insulin secretion and resistance; decreasing sugar and carbohydrates intake helps to reduce insulin levels. These strategies have led to lower insulin levels, the critical factor of the obesity problem.

One consequence of childhood obesity is that it could lead to adult obesity and its future health problems like heart disease. Childhood obesity can be considered a predictor of increased mortality. It is imperative to find that obesity is a reversible risk factor. Thus, children who are overweight or obese and become a standard weight as an adult, have the same percentages of probability to those adults who have never been overweight.

In Britain, about one-third of the children between the ages of 2 and 15 who are overweight or obese, will lead to a massive cost of £5.1 billion to the National Health Service. So, Britain's failure to eat a balanced diet will cost the NHS a fortune. Parents should start helping in the fight against child obesity by educating and refusing to give their children sweet treats.

Treating childhood obesity means more than just changing food/diet and physical activity habits. It is also imperative to address the emotional and social impact that overweight children can carry on their quality of life. Unfortunately, the stigma in our society about obesity is still high. A stigma is associated with binge eating, social isolation, reduced physical activity, and additional weight gain over time. These can all exacerbate obesity and make healthy behaviour changes hard. So, it is vital to keep it positive. We all know that making a change is hard, and patients will have difficulties initially meeting some of their objectives. But, we can learn from these challenges and go from there. It is also crucial that these children get the support that they need by the paediatricians who can speak to children and parents about their weight, and that they are supportive and encouraging, instead of sounding unintentionally judgemental.

# 3.2 - How does junk food destroy our children's health?

The eating habits that you are creating in your life can have a huge impact on your children. I'm talking about the impact you can have on your children by the food you consume. You are teaching these habits to your loved ones, and the way you approach food will be in their memories forever. It has amazed me that food is what makes us who we are, and yet we take it so lightly.

If you have children, eating junk food can be harmful to their health, and it should also never be a reward. We really need to change our habits and our mind-set.

The problem with fast foods is that they contain delicious ingredients like salt, fat, and sugars, and their taste draws children and non-children like a magnet. Since the evolution of human beings, our brain is hard-wired to crave high-calorie food as a mechanism of survival. So, when we see, smell, and eat fast food, our body releases chemicals and neurotransmitters (dopamine is secreted) which are responsible for this excitement and pleasure. Then, due to this effect, the child has a lack of control and the brain desires more and more junk food.

One study was done in schools about junk food consumption and the performance of children in reading and maths.

The results showed that the pupils who consumed junk food five times per week scored much lower in math and reading. On the other hand, studies show that eating fruits, vegetables, nuts, and fish are right for your children. They contain high levels of antioxidants and healthy fats. This contributes to a good function of the brain. Thus, the consumption of fast food lacks those nutritional values and, therefore, can lead to lack of concentration and a risk of depression.

The consequences of obesity in children can include having a higher risk of developing chronic illnesses in their adult life, such as type 2 diabetes, heart problems, or cancer. Also, studies showed that these children are more likely to be bullied, as they have a low self-esteem. And, yet, the unfortunate thing is that children are not taught in school about the importance of which foods to eat and which healthy habits they should follow.

Furthermore, the intake of junk food tends to replace other more nutritional meals. When children eat biscuits, crisps, or sweets, they do not usually consume hardly any fruits or vegetables, which will reduce their vitamin C and fibre. This lack of fibre may lead to abdominal pain, discomfort, and constipation. Also, sweetened beverages and fast food contain high levels of sugar. Therefore, it is associated with fluctuations in children's blood glucose, which can contribute to making them sleepy, irritable, and edgy.

Studies revealed that consuming sugary drinks or fruit juice during dinnertime, even if only twice a week, can affect children's sleep and wake-up cycle. The content of caffeine from sodas react as stimulants, and this makes them stay awake longer.

Research showed that around forty percent of parents reported that they often give into their children's demands for fast food. If your child's continuous whining has led you to swerve into a drive-through to get your children chips and burgers, you are not alone.

But, the next time you suggest getting dinner on the go, think twice with regard to the impact it will have on your kids.

When your child bites into a chip, her brain-reward system gets activated and dopamine gets secreted. This neurotransmitter is responsible for this pleasure and excitement, your child will have no control, and her brain will demand more and more.

Scientific studies revealed that once children started eating junk food, they ingested more calories and fewer nutrients during the day. For instance, on days when children consumed junk food, they consumed 309 calories. On days when they ate at home, they only consumed 126 calories.

Health practitioners discovered that, in the long run, consumption of fast food clogs arteries, and this effect begins on the first day. Studies showed that this happened immediately, after just one—that's right, one—fast food meal. This is very scary.

Unfortunately, childhood obesity is a huge problem that the world faces nowadays. The rates of childhood obesity have risen to alarming levels in the USA. A proposal was made to simply and easily bring the rate of obesity in childhood down. The proposal was to serve water with school lunch instead of fizzy and carbonated juices and drinks. It concluded that it was better to encourage students to drink water and not fizzy drinks with high sugar. By undertaking this strategy, it will help prevent nearly half a million young people in the USA from becoming overweight or developing diabetes or other health conditions.

Unfortunately, fast food can be very addictive, and children used to spicy junk foods may have some trouble adjusting their palates to relatively blander healthy foods. So, the best thing you can do for your children in the first place is not to give them junk food at all. Thus, if you teach them well in what and how to eat since their childhood, it is more likely they will go for the right and healthier choice!

## 3:3 - What habits do we need to encourage in our children for a healthier life?

Sadly, our habits have changed from over a decade ago. For instance, in the past, a coach used to provide oranges during break time in a sports event. Nowadays, they are replaced with lollies or fruit chews. What happened? I am concerned this unhealthy snack does not send the right message. Everyone should know by now that the nutritional value of lollies or sweets is zero, and they are merely empty sugar calories (artificial flavour and colour), and this only contributes to a weight gain.

My main concern is that the rewards and prizes at sports games are fast food vouchers from team sponsors. Our children are bombarded with junk food marketing, and they are being exposed to unhealthy food advertisements daily. This is scary, because, in the end, we all contribute to normalising fast food, and this promotes a society that normalises obesity and encourages behaviours that cause weight gain when we all know this it is detrimental to our health.

Therefore, we must not set up a habit of 'junk food as reward' mentality. We must take every opportunity to inspire our children to make nutritious food choices that set them up for life.

As for me, I am passionate about this topic. I care for children, and it breaks my heart to see children so young, less than a toddler's age, eating crisps and drinking sweetened drinks. We live in a wealthy country where we can have all the food of the world, and yet parents give their children such quality poor food. That is why I have written this book and shared my message. So, please think twice every time you eat or when you feed your children.

This has gone too far, why do we allow this to happen? Let's be responsible people and stop blaming others or society or the government about our lousy choice of eating patterns. Let's make a difference by undertaking good habits and avoid eating junk food. Let's have a rich diet full of vitamins and proteins that help us to rejuvenate our cells, organs, and body system in general.

Let me introduce my friend and her son Luis. Luis is a ten-year-old child who became overweight and then obese. He also became part of the obesity statistics. But Luis is not only a statistic, or a number; he is a human being, a real person, with feelings and emotions about being overweight.

His mother always tries her best to give him fresh, good food, but as a single mother, it was not easy if you had a full-time job. Luis' mother sometimes got home very tired with no energy to cook. So, she usually bought the takeaways on her way home. It was an effortless and comfortable way to provide some dinner to her son. The fact is that the majority of the takeaways are high in fats and sugars. Mother and son noted that they were putting on weight more and more as the months passed by. We all know how cruel the children can be at school. Luis felt excluded and lonely in school. He became depressed, and he only wanted to eat. Yes, I know; it's a vicious circle, isn't it?

Luis received help from health professionals, and in the end, he managed to lose a lot of weight, but not before losing a lot of battles. He had the help of a paediatrician, dietician, and a psychologist. They helped him physically and mentally.. He was determined to transform his bad eating habits to healthier habits. His transformation to implement new practices would help him to get fitter and feel good about himself. The first habit that he achieved was to avoid any processed food and stick to the fresh and natural food. By applying this, he couldn't go wrong! We always need to remember to teach good habits to our children, starting at a very early age.

To help your children learn healthy habits, it's all about setting a good example! It is paramount that parents lead by example and their children will reflect their habits. The parents are the ones who look after their children, and they are a driving force for their children's health. One good practice is as simple as getting families to eat around the table, and not in front of the television.

A fundamental habit of emphasising is the importance of the family meal times. This is critical to help the behaviours, attitudes, and conversations when eating together as a family. Thus, it can have a primary influence towards shaping your child's relationship with food. For children, parents are the role models, and children like to imitate what they hear, perceive, and see. Consequently, it is vital to remember that the knowledge and habits children obtain from the dinner table are likely to remain with them throughout life.

We need to tell our children that health is more important than looks. This involves encouraging children to feel good, to have a balanced diet, and to be healthy, rather than focussing on losing weight or avoiding weight gain. Again, it is the mind-set that we want to inculcate in our children.

The implementation of a simple habit—like serving water with school lunches—can contribute considerably to reduce the rates of childhood and adult obesity. Research showed the impact that even small steps can lead to encouraging healthy body weight. So, the habits we develop as children, as young as two or three years old, can have a significant influence on the behaviour we carry into adulthood. This is why identifying a healthy lifestyle when we are very young is vital to preventing obesity and other illnesses in the future.

So, during a child's mealtime, the best alternative drinks are water or low fat dairy. If your child does not like water, or finds it boring, then get creative. Keep a water pitcher in the refrigerator and flavour it with the fresh cut of cucumbers, lemons, oranges, or berries. Let your children get their favourite water bottle.

For our body health, water is a vital nutrient. Furthermore, water is also considered a natural appetite suppressant, so it helps you keep a healthy weight.

Another good habit to implement in our children for a healthier life is the reduction of sugar-sweetened beverages. A study done between 7 and 11 year old children showed that the reduction of sugar-sweetened beverages is an amazingly useful strategy for preventing obesity in childhood.

Sugary drinks like juices and sodas and their consumption have contributed to rising levels of obesity. For example, a 20-ounce soda has approximately 17 teaspoons of sugar, which is the equivalent of roughly 240 calories, and it also triggers the hormone insulin. If your child consumes this every single day, it can bring nothing but OBESITY.

The consumption of this amount of calories in liquid format will not make an individual feel full. Therefore, they won't compensate for the calorie intake by eating less. Moreover, studies have shown that sugary drinks might affect the increased risk for leptin resistance as well. Leptin is also known as the starvation hormone. High levels of leptin can tell your brain that you are full and your hunger will go away.

Parents have the main role in convincing their children to avoid sweetened drinks, but it won't be easy, as sugary drinks are everywhere.

To reduce the consumption of sugary drinks, parents should eliminate them as an option and have another alternative at home. When at a social event, the right message is that these drinks are only for once in a while. The vital aspect of this is to reduce the need for sweetness. This is similar to adults; once they go without it for a long enough time, they lose the desire to have it.

Instead of the sweet snacks your children are used to, a good habit and an excellent alternative are fresh fruits or vegetables, such as pears, mandarins, berries, cherry tomatoes, or carrots. Dried fruits and nuts are also great for a balanced and healthy diet. And please promote drinking water for re-hydrating, and staying away from sports drinks, sodas, or other sugary drinks.

Our body (hair, muscles, organs, brain, nails, bones, etc.) is made of every single cell of what we eat. What we eat affects our concentration, our physical and psychological development, our behaviour, and our learning capacity. Let's encourage nutrient-dense foods to help our children to grow and develop to their full potential. Make a radical transformation in your life that helps you to feel good and amazing about yourself and your children.

# Chapter 4:
# Obesity and Reward Food

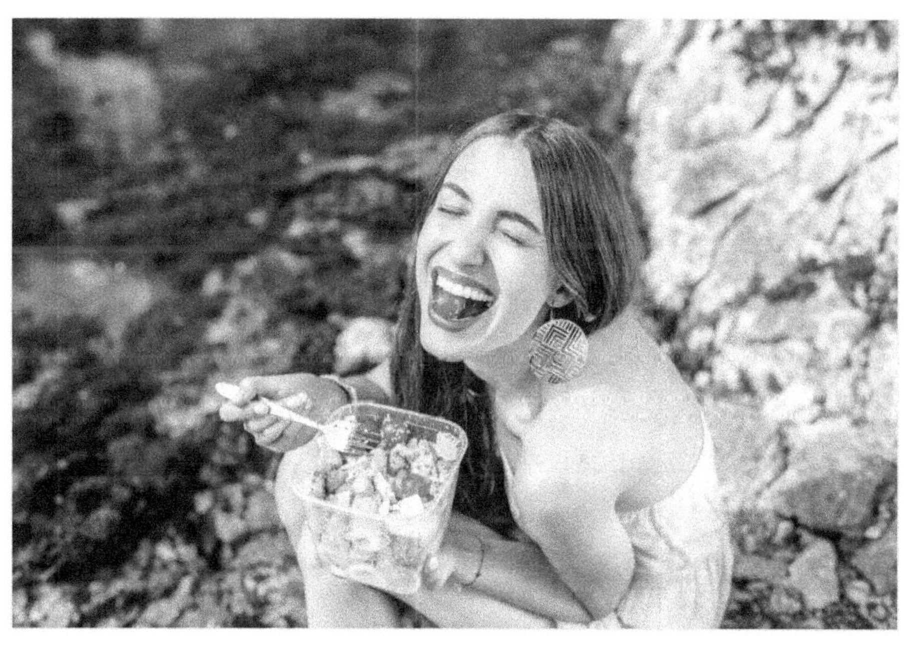

Healthy foods help the fight against obesity

# 4.1 - What is obesity and reward food?

Obesity is a simple term used when somebody is grossly overweight or has a lot of body fat. It has become quite a common problem over the last decade. The number of adults rated as being obese in the United Kingdom (UK) is around one in every four adults.

A body mass index (BMI) greater than 30 is considered obese.

It is very worrying that the rates of obesity in adulthood and childhood rose in not only the UK but also all around the world. Policy makers and researchers search for new ways to reverse these trends.

In the United States, an increased incidence of adult obesity is on the rise. In the Western society, some of the primary causes of obesity are due to reduced physical activity leading to a sedentary lifestyle and a surplus of processed food, junk food, and soda drinks. The variety of fast food and its hyper-palatable ingredients contribute to activating dopamine-rewarding centres leading to over-consumption of this kind of food. Hyper-palatable foods and their increased availability promote addictive and compulsive eating leading to weight gain. The overabundance of food seems to aid in food addiction and specifically foods rich in sugars and other carbohydrates.

There are a significant number of people that are addicted to sugar and starch. Highly refined carbohydrates in the forms of sweets, breads, rice, crackers, cereals, or flour can lead to a blood sugar roller coaster ride. Thus, carbohydrate craving is associated with carbohydrates, insulin, and appetite.

While eating carbohydrates, our insulin rises, which then diminishes our blood sugar. The increase of insulin leads to weight gain. After eating and filling up on this kind of food, the blood sugar rises quickly and then plummets, leaving individuals cranky, shaky, and ravenous. Without realising what was going on, their hunger would lead them to fill up again and again on low fat, highly refined carbs, such as fat-free cookies, rice cakes, bagels, and so on. With the habit of eating this kind of food, most people ended up fat, unhappy, overfed, and undernourished, because they didn't know how to fuel themselves properly. More and more people are sensitive to sugar and starch, and this is the main reason that has led to an explosion of obesity, diabetes, and other chronic diseases.

For people who are sugar/starch sensitive, it is about doing what they can to maintain their blood sugar levels. Understanding how blood sugar and insulin work in our body can be confusing. So, to put it in simple terms: think of a very slow, steady drip from a faucet. When you blast your body with a lot of sugar/starch, you flood your bloodstream with sugars, so it has to release insulin to divert all that excess out of your bloodstream and into your cells. Unfortunately, in order to compensate, your body usually ends up releasing too much insulin, which causes your blood sugar to drop too low and that leads to hunger signals and another sugar surge, where the cycle repeats itself again and again. Thus, these continuous ups and downs are hard on your body, and they can lead to obesity, insulin sensitivity, diabetes, and heart disease.

The majority of researchers and nutritionists agreed that fats from junk food triggered the brain to want more food, which, of course, leads to obesity.

People don't want to be obese for the sake of being overweight, and diets usually fail because hunger overrides other motivations.

When we eat food, there is an element called *palatability* or *reward*, which provokes us to eat more. Foods with high palatability contribute to overeating and getting fat. Why can't we just blame palatability or reward?

Research in Sidney revealed that junk food could reprogram our brain into having an increased desire for unhealthy choices.

Let me tell you some food facts about junk food that might convince you to eat healthier foods:

The term junk food has been with us since the 1960s, but within the last two decades, it has become very popular. Research demonstrated that the high consumption of junk food is associated with the increase in heart disease, obesity, hypertension, and certain cancers.

There is an essential factor that influences our lives, and that is television. It is a proven fact that almost 80% of all food adverts that are on the air on Saturday during children's shows are for junk food.

Junk food manufacturers continue to try to hook people (and mainly children) to consume junk food. It was the American snack, Crackerjack, that became one of the first food products to use toys to target junk food to children.

At 23 billion dollars annually, the US is the leader of junk food sales in the world. And, candy sales continue to increase, despite concerns over junk food and obesity. More than two billion dollars in candy is sold for Halloween alone, more than any other holiday in America, which leads to Halloween being the unhealthiest and fattest food holiday.

The most popular junk food in the world is French fries. One portion of these chips has approximately 600 calories of carbohydrates, which triggers our insulin levels. But, instead of staving off your hunger, it will do the opposite and leave you wanting more.

The obesity epidemic looks unstoppable. Studies have revealed that globally approximately 1 billion adults are overweight of which 475 million are obese. Obesity is a complex multifactorial condition. Statistics show that more than one-third of adults in the United States are obese. Obesity is leading to approximately 300,000 deaths every year, and it is pointing to the second leading cause of preventable death in the U.S. Furthermore, obesity is causing a burden to the healthcare system and in obesity-related morbidities in the U.S.

In 2015, approximately 58% of women and 68% of men in England were overweight or obese. If the obesity epidemic carries on like this, the next 35 years will bankrupt the health care system, the government, and us. But what is relevant is the cost in human lives, and any human suffering is unmeasurable. Many will suffer badly and die needlessly.

Health experts claim that obesity is rising in Africa and, consequently, the number of cases of diabetes is widely increasing as well. In Africa, children with an overweight or obese problem have doubled since 1990, rising from 5.4 million to 10.3 million. Diet and diabetes cannot be separated. With the increasing number of individuals suffering from non-communicable diseases such as cancer and diabetes, calls to eat healthy food have been rising. It is essential that people start with healthy lifestyles/habits from an early age.

The World Health Organisation's (WHO) statistics reveal that in developing countries in Africa and across the globe, the diabetes population will double by 2040. Health professionals report that the epidemic of diabetes in this continent is rising mainly because of the combined effects of rapid urbanization, environmental changes, changing eating habits, and an increase in life expectancy.

In the last few years, diabetes has turned into one of the most massive epidemics of the twenty-first century, ahead of AIDS and HIV. Health experts encourage people to watch their eating habits and their exercise patterns. Sadly, diabetes is a significant risk factor for other terrible diseases, such as heart condition, kidney failure, and stroke.

## 4.2 - What are the causes of obesity?

There are thousands of books and information about obesity and weight gain or weight loss that you can use, and yet there is still a complete lack of a theoretical framework for understanding obesity. There are many theories that can be quite simplistic and often take into account only one element, such as 'excess dietary fat causes obesity,' 'hardly any physical activity causes obesity,' 'excess carbohydrates cause obesity,' or 'excess calories cause obesity.'

The other major problem for understanding obesity is the evidence-based or short-term studies when obesity normally takes decades to develop. As obesity is a long-term condition, short-term studies may not be fully informative. For years, we seemed to find the solution to obesity by implementing the method of eating less and moving more with the understanding that the ultimate solution was to eat fewer calories. But, if that is the solution, why do we have so much obesity?

In human history, we were not that obsessed with calories, and obesity was a rare condition. As civilisations developed, obesity appeared. Speculations of the cause of this condition targeted refined carbohydrates, like sugar and starches.

Let me tell you a story, a real story, of a man in the nineteenth century who never had problems with his weight in his twenties.

But, throughout his thirties, he noted that he was gaining weight at the rate of one or two pounds per year. By the time he reached the age of sixty years old, he was obese, and he wanted to have a winning formula to lose weight. He was so distressed that he sought advice on weight loss from his physicians. First, he tried to eat less, but that failed as it left him even hungrier. Second, he tried to exercise more by rowing along a river. While he was improving his physical fitness, he failed badly at losing weight, because he had a bigger appetite after rowing.

Finally, he tried a new approach, with the idea that starchy and sugary foods were fattening. He avoided all beer, potatoes, cakes, sweets, and breads that were the major part of his diet (today, it is known as low in refined carbohydrates). It was by following this eating approach that he lost weight and, not only that, he kept it off for the rest of his days. He wrote a pamphlet about his experience in gaining weight that he believed resulted from eating too many fattening carbohydrates.

From that century, the standard treatment for obesity was to implement a low refined carbohydrate diet. By the 1950s it became fairly standard advice. If you asked people what caused obesity, they would not mention calories. Instead, they would say to you to stop eating starches and sugars.

So, what happened? How did this obsession of calories in and calories out start? In the 1960s, many people died from heart attacks, in the U.S. in particular. Dietary fat was thought to raise the levels of cholesterol, a fatty component that is believed to contribute to the heart condition. Soon, health professionals began to advocate lower-fat diets. And, since then, the demonization of dietary fat started in earnest.

Thus, the stipulation of the dietary guidelines for Americans by the American Heart Association (AHA) and the foods that we should eat every single day were bread, potatoes, and pasta. These were the same foods that we had previously avoided to stay thin. The AHA declared an Eating Plan for Healthy Americans. And it was that we should eat six or more servings of pasta, cereals, and starchy vegetables that are low in fat and cholesterol. They also declared we should drink carbonated soda drinks or fruit punches. Well done American Heart Association! With all our focus on fat, we took our eyes off the ball. Everything was about reducing cholesterol and reducing fat, and nobody was focusing on sugar. Food manufacturers added more sugars in processed food for flavour. The increase of refined grain consumption went up forty-five percent. Thus, people ate more and more low-fat pastas or starches, not broccoli or kale.

In spite of the implementation of the AHA diet of low fat, the rate of obesity did not decrease; it kept rising.

Thus, a massive increase in obesity started when the AHA decided to change the American diet to a low-fat, high-carbohydrate, and sugary diet. Was it a mere coincidence?

Studies revealed that the causes of obesity are not only the consuming of more calories; it's the kind of calories we're ingesting, especially those in sugary and carbohydrate foods. Researchers found that our hormonal metabolism, in particular the insulin hormone, continues to lead the epidemic of obesity. A high level of insulin in our body helps to increase weight.

For decades, health professionals kept telling us to eat a healthy, reduced-calorie diet and exercise regularly. Throughout all these years, they sent us the same message again and again, but nobody was losing weight. This sounds like it was not that simple to reduce weight.

Researchers found that there is much more to it than just cutting the caloric intake and doing more exercises to decrease the body weight. They believe it is much more about the hormonal metabolism stereotype.

Studies showed that obesity causes can also be associated with genes. The inheritance aspect can be one of the causes of obesity. But the fact is that being overweight or obese can also be related to a variety of elements from an inability to regulate appetite to a malfunction in energy expenditure. Studies revealed information about the genetic data of a large number of individuals where the researchers identified around fourteen genetic variations related to the obesity epidemic and body mass index (BMI).

The contribution of two hundred and fifty research institutions was taken in a massive study from around the world. Researchers highlighted fourteen specific genetic variations, how most of them were identified as playing a fundamental role in the control of body weight, and how these genes were considered as new targets for obesity research.

One of the discoveries was a copy variation in a gene called MC4R. The gene variant, found in almost 1 in 5,000 people, affects the production of a protein that regulates appetite and results in carriers weighing an average of 15 lb (6.8 kg) heavier than those without the genetic variant. Another discovery revealed two variants in the GIPR gene, found in about 1 in 400 people, corresponding with an average of 4.5 lb (2 kg) more weight than non-carriers.

The fact is many people find it challenging to make healthy choices in an environment where food and drinks are made with so much salt, sugar, and fat; are heavily promoted; cheap; and widely available.

Unfortunately, there are many misleading messages out there about diet, food, and nutrition. The food industry, and the way they sell their products, is very much based on a clever use of marketing and buzzwords on food and drink products, which make us believe some food products are healthy when, in reality, they're not.

Food companies have that tendency of marketing products as healthy, even though they might not be a healthier option in all aspects. For instance, we may be encouraged to eat a product that contains fruit and looks healthy, but in fact, it may not contain much fruit at all.

Now, about potato chips: medical scientists corroborated that potato chips, as well as French fries and other deep fried goodies (wings or chicken fingers), can be the cause of different diseases in North America. So, think twice before slipping into a drive-thru for some crispy-greasy satisfaction, and consider the danger you can put on your rectum, prostate, breasts, bladder, and colon. The primary factor of the risk of these conditions comes from acrylamide, a carcinogen produced during the in-depth fried cooking process.  A healthier alternative would be to bake the potatoes at home. Bake them in the oven until crispy.

With regard to the refined white carbohydrates: there are few of them! In fact, nearly the whole supermarket is full of them! Cookies, pre-packed chips, white bread, white rice, pasta, cakes, bakery products, breakfast cereals, and pretty much every single snack food on the market all have one thing in common—they all contain wheat flour. The property of these products is that they digest very fast into simple sugars, leading to blood sugar levels that spike and drop quickly in a wave of irritability and mid-day snack attacks. Nutritionists found that a starchy addition is related to type 2 diabetes, high blood pressure, inflammatory diseases (arthritis), and weight gain.

Hot dogs. What do I mean by hot dogs? I refer to any cured, smoked, or salted meat that is full of chemical preservatives. Nutritionists reported that hot dogs are awful for your health and suggested they have a warning label like cigarettes have. Studies revealed that the regular consumption of hot dogs could heighten the risk of colorectal cancer by approximately 21%. To be sure you get chemical-free hot dogs and sausages, buy them from your local butcher. Once again, just because it's in the market, doesn't mean it's good for you.

The essential element that affects the metabolisation of fat is the relative proportions of fats, proteins, and carbohydrates in the diet.

When we eat, we have a reward and gratification associated with our food intake. The consumption of food releases dopamine production. Dopamine is a hormone that activates the reward and pleasure centres of the brain. Thus, an individual can repeatedly eat a specific food to experience this positive feeling of gratification.

Also, studies found that mood disorders and our emotions are often related to abnormal feeding behaviour. For instance, anxiety is a comorbidity of obesity. There is a tendency in those who are obese to have a higher risk of suffering depression. This depression involves a higher level of both endocrine and metabolic conditions due to the poor choice or selection of food intake. They usually prefer to consume comfort foods as a means to alleviate their negative feelings.

## 4.3 - What habits can we implement to stop getting fat?

As we all know, losing weight is not easy. If it were, we would not have millions of diets or products. Thus, the smallest tips, or the implementation of habits, can make a big difference in weight loss plans.

Here are some of the new habits that you can implement to help you keep your weight down.

Get into the habit of using colour plates that contrast the foods you usually eat, so the portions will looks bigger.

I encourage you to get into the habit of fasting one or two meals per week. Apart from keeping you in good shape, it is a very healthy way to repair the cells of your body. This is not nearly as hard as it sounds. It becomes one of the simplest things to do, doing nothing—no shopping, no cooking, no washing. This method of eating is about implementing occasional fasts (periods when you can drink water, but skip one or two meals of your day) into your regular eating habits.

When I fast, I drink a glass of water every hour or two. I recommend you do the same. If you are new to fasting, I encourage you to try it, as it is not as complicated or hard as you may think. During a lot of your hours of fasting, you will be sleeping, plus you will still have two meals on each day. Make it a goal to do it. Start once a month, then twice a month, and so on. Fasting is an eating pattern that burns calories. The way it works is that your insulin increases when your body processes food; therefore, it is difficult for your body to burn fat. However, when your body fasts, the insulin decreases, and, consequently, it is easier for your body to burn fat.

Mindfulness is a powerful instrument in all aspects of your lives, and this includes how you eat. Simply pay more attention to your food when you eat. A good tip is that when you eat do not do anything else but eat. Look closely at what you are having, eat more slowly, and between bites put your spoon, fork, and fingers down. With these habits, you will eat less without really noticing.

Take a simple action to design your behaviour. Ensure that your environment will help you to lose weight, instead of feeling guilty or lacking motivation. It's all about designing your behaviour.

One good tip is to order sauces or dressings on the side.

Moreover, the NHS digital report revealed that only 26% of adults ate the recommended five portions of fruit or vegetables a day in 2015.

A spokesman for the Obesity Health Alliance, a coalition of more than forty health charities, campaign groups, and medical colleges, reported: As waistlines increase, so do the chances of developing life-threatening conditions like type 2 diabetes, heart disease, and cancer, putting a further strain on our already overstretched health service.

Once again, this is a good reminder of the exact reason that we need measures like the sugar reduction programme and the soft drink industry levy to help us create a healthier environment for all.

Public Health England (PHE) reports and pushes the food industries to tackle obesity by shrinking chocolate bars and sweets. The PHE is urging the food industry to help fight obesity by cutting 20% of the sugar from the main snacks and foods that children eat.

The confectionery industry claims that removing sugar and keeping the taste would be difficult. The PHE had a proposal to this sector, and it is that they could make the change by shrinking the size of the chocolate bars and sweets they sell. The targets are cakes, pastries, ice cream, breakfast cereal, biscuits, yoghurts, puddings, and sweet spreads.

If we are going to be serious about changing the nation's sweet tooth, the food industry as a whole needs to commit to the government's very welcome 20% reduction target and take collective responsibility for a change.

First however, food experts make suggestions to the government, but it has rejected a number of the recommendations, such as a rigorous control on supermarkets selling unhealthy food and drinks to children.

To perform well at work on a daily basis, the best habit I have is to make sure that I eat accordingly, with good fuel, not just any fuel. My mind and physical body have to be in harmony. Fresh and natural foods are the best to feed your body.

I know we live in a society where we are full of distractions, so much so that we have forgotten how to eat correctly. But then, if it is not the most valuable thing, what is it? I always understood that health is the first thing one must have, not money or a career. If one does have good health, the rest comes second. Start seeing yourself as a piece of engineering with a high standard of performance. So, the most valuable thing to do is to look after your body, and your mind, to help you to be happy and healthy, and energetic and feel amazing.

So, my million-dollar question is: why then, do we let the food industries and their marketing ruin our lives with fast food that takes us to the graveyard earlier that we are supposed to go?

Enough is enough. Instead of taking a cocktail of tablets, think about eating fresh and nutritious foods as a new medicine, a new therapy to help you to have a fantastic life.

Meet my friend Julie. She is an overweight lady. Her body mass index (BMI) is around 29.2. She is a housewife, and she has four children. About her health, there was nothing specific, but being overweight was her worse enemy. She knew that being overweight could bring complications or diseases during her lifetime. She also had antecedents of her father suffering from type 2 diabetes, and, sadly, he died due to complications of his illness.

Julie was worried about her father's diabetic condition, and the possibility that she could get it as well. Then, she had a routine check-up with her doctor, and she was told that she was borderline about developing diabetes. Julie was very concerned about this possibility. So, she cut out a lot of biscuits, cakes, pies, and pizza. To her amazement, she was not only losing weight, but she also had better-controlled blood sugar levels in her body.

She was delighted with the results. She realised that high sugary products and simple carbohydrate foods produce an increase in the insulin hormone. Thus, the existence of an increase in the insulin hormone resulted in an increase in her weight. She was very pleased with her results at the beginning, but then the temptations became stronger than her willingness to give up the biscuits and cakes, even though it was for her own good.

I encouraged her not to buy this kind of food, but she seemed to have the perfect excuse, according to her. She has grandchildren, and she would not deprive her grandchildren of eating biscuits or cakes. I asked her why not? I told her: You are not doing them any favours by feeding your grandchildren junk food. In fact, it is quite the opposite. You're turning them into sugar addicts, and you are putting unnecessary weight in your grandchildren's bodies that, in the long run, could lead to diabetes or obesity. So, what eating habits do you want to follow?

My friend, Julie is a clear example of how challenging it is to break bad habits. She thought it was alright treating her grandchildren with sweets and cakes, and unfortunately, she is not alone. We grew up in a society where, if you are a good boy or girl, treats with biscuits or lollipops are the norm.

This society and the food industries sell us anything they want as long as they can get their profit. And the truth is that the processed foods on sale in the supermarkets are not good for us.

We must become fully conscious in our mind that what we want to put in our mouth and, most importantly, what we want to put in our children's mouths is of good nutritional quality. They are our future generations, and we want a generation as healthy as possible and not rotten from diseases and detrimental eating patterns.

We just cannot only blame the government, the policy makers, and the food industries about the rapid increase of the obesity epidemic. We also need to take responsibility for it too.

# Chapter 5:
# Fasting

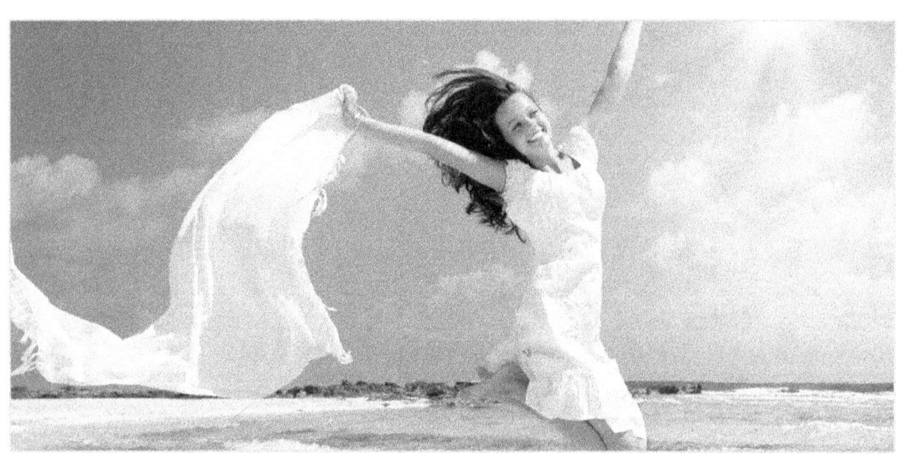

Fasting helps to sharpen your brain and your body

# 5.1 - Why fasting?

The reason for this topic is because I believe that fasting is good for you, and it is an amazing habit. I've been doing it for a few years now, and it provides good health results. I feel healthier now than previously, before doing any fasting.

Fasting is a voluntary way of not eating, and the health benefits have been proven. There's a quote by Friedrich Nietzsche: That which does not kill us, makes us stronger. While starvation is bad for you, fasting is good for you.

I started fasting around five years ago with my colleague, Wendy. We did the intermittent fasting method. Intermittent fasting became very popular after Dr Michael Mosley's filmed documentary about fasting in his Horizon programme, *Eat, Fast and Live Longer* in 2012.

While Wendy started fasting as an eating plan way of losing weight, I did it because I could see the health benefits of doing it. I think our body needs a break from eating and that gives my cells the chance to repair and grow. After fasting, I feel amazing, and I think it's one of the best decisions that I've ever made. It became a habit, and now I'm doing it without realising it. I must admit that when I started, it was a bit challenging. But, with time and practice, fasting became a costume, a lifestyle.

I do not have problems with my weight, but I recognise the importance of keeping a healthy body and mind. And, according to medical evidence, this can be achieved with better results through intermittent fasting. This means I choose one or two days of each week to fast with a restriction in calories of 500 g, split by having a small breakfast and a small dinner. The intention is to keep twelve hours fasting between a small breakfast and a small dinner. I do not have fixed days to do this, but mainly Mondays and Thursdays. I make sure that I fast one or two days of every week, most of the time.

If you want to do a favour to your body and feel amazing afterwards, try intermittent fasting. It is a more manageable and sustainable way of keeping fit and healthy than any other eating regime. Please, think about it. Your body is designed to fast; we are the product of feast and fast. We have evolved from our ancestors of the feast or famine times. Humanity was evolved when food was scarce. Religions like Greek Orthodox Christian or Ramadan fast on a regular basis as a part of their lifestyle. Fasting mimics our evolution more accurately than three meals a day, which is how modern humans have been shaped.

We have been told for decades that we must eat at least three meals per day, then some years later, we were told to have a snack in between meals, and then we were told that we must never skip meals, and we must watch our calories. And do not forget to exercise more as well, of course. Nowadays, we are eating all the time, and we are rarely hungry. And by default, we all carry on this way of eating. But it has been shown, that more and more obesity levels have risen, and more than ever, we are suffering from metabolic syndrome problems, such as diabetes.

This message has been in our lives throughout the years, but it doesn't work. Fasting is an ancient idea but a modern method. Most of the time, we are dissatisfied with our body and our health, and fasting helps us to connect with ourselves. Scientists found that fasting is a powerful tool, that it can benefit us with weight loss, disease resistance, and longevity.

I'm not talking about eating/dieting regimes that are normally drastic, where, at the beginning, you lose weight and then you lose faith. And those dieting regimes can be too complicated to implement, or too hard to follow, and doomed to fail. Research has shown about the positive impact of intermittent fasting on our bodies, and the great impact of fasting on cancer, and its efficacy on chemotherapy and radiotherapy.

Medical and scientific evidence was extensive, and the compelling medical community was positive about intermittent fasting (IF). They found out about a life extension by focussing on calorie restriction (CR) and fasting. Fasting cut the range of diseases like diabetes or cancer. It's not just a diet; it's a sustainable and realistic strategy for long-term health gains.

As individuals with our biochemical profile, we do not have the willpower or desire to live in a reduced-calorie state every single day. Instead, we can go for intermittent fasting, which is to eat less but only for one or two days every week.

There are many forms of intermittent fasting. Some examples are: nothing to eat for 24 hours; a single meal every day; have 5/7 (five days eat normally and then two days of a reduction in calories); eat 500 calories, 250 for breakfast and 250 for supper; or 12 hours fasting as a stretch. With intermittent fasting, you can choose to fast any days you would like to. Once you get used to it, it becomes an amazing habit. I embraced fasting, and it became part of my daily life. I do it automatically; I do it because I know it is good for my body, for my brain, and for my persona.

## 5.2 - What are the benefits of fasting?

Our hunter-gatherer ancestors did not eat four or five times a day. Sometimes, they would have had a feast in times of plenty, and then sometimes they would fast for a certain period, as they couldn't find any food. Bearing this in mind, it makes sense that our body's cells could perform well under the harsh conditions of feast or famine. They searched for food most of the time; they hunted for food. Their genes evolved in an environment of scarcity.

About two decades ago, we weren't used to snacking between meals. Now, it seems a normal thing to do, and it has become a bad eating habit.

It was a suggestion from the medical professionals that snacking was a good idea, as it could contribute to reducing your appetite. It was also said that it was implemented by snack manufactures or faddish diet books. But, snacking does not lead you to eat less. Studies revealed that approximately in the

1970s, the standard of not eating was four and half hours between meals, now it's hardly three hours.

There are also arguments within the medical establishment that eating is better in small meals, as it is less likely you will eat too much or get hungry and gorge on junk food, for instance. But, this way of eating led us to eat more, and we consumed more calories in comparison to the last twenty years.

I think we eat more because it has become a habit, because the food is there, from boredom, or we're afraid our hunger will build and build, and it will become intolerable. But, hunger pangs do pass away. Once you overcome hunger, you no longer fear it.

As for me, fasting helps me to sharpen my senses and my brain. When I started, I was a bit concerned that I may feel faint or dizzy. But it turned out fine, and I have experienced that our body can be very adaptable. Do you know that many athletes fast during their training?

Let me explain in simple terms how our biology operates at the cellular level. For example, exercise damages your muscles. It forms tears and rips in the body's response to the stressor (damaged muscle cells). By doing repairs, it makes your muscles stronger. The health benefits of intermittent fasting are that scientific studies have revealed that whilst fasting your blood sugar levels are dropped. Thus, during fasting, our cells have to work harder to utilise other forms of energy, like glycogen and ketone bodies that act as a sort of energy instead of glucose, and this is just one part of the body's repair.

Thanks to scientific evidence, intermittent fasting has revealed the reduction of IGF-1 in our bodies. IGF-1 stands for Insulin-like Growth Factor 1. It is a protein that forms part of the human body that is encoded by the IGF1 gene. IGF-1 keeps our cells active when we are young. However, in our adult life, too many cells of this factor accelerate life, leading to a higher risk of suffering from cancer and heart disease.

Thus, benefits of IGF-1 reduction mean that we have a better chance to fight if any signs of cancer cells occur, as there are genes that switch on to repair and protect, in response to the stressor (cancer cells).

When we age, we approach a higher risk of age-related diseases like diabetes and cancer. Normally, people who fast do not have those diseases and live a long life. The main reason for fasting is that it gives us extraordinary health benefits. It helps to improve your brain function, it decreases insulin sensitivity (which should reduce your risk of obesity), and it helps to reduce cognitive ailments, like Alzheimer's. Also, it contributes to keeping your insulin levels low when you start eating again, which, at the same time, lowers your risk of deadly diseases.

Fasting also helps to improve your immune system, it helps your body maintain lean muscle, and it helps in weight loss and longevity, thanks to continuous repair performance of the cells. The Romans did practice fasting by doing one day in four, or one day in three, and it revealed results of a longer life. So, to summarise, the primary objective of intermittent fasting is weight loss and better health, two sides of the same page.

Furthermore, studies on mice showed the value of fasting. In mice that they did not fast, the longevity record was an average of two years. However, in those mice that they fasted, their longevity was around four years, and the mice stayed healthy, and they didn't show any signs of having diabetes or cancer diseases. The autopsy results concluded that they died due to old age, a natural death.

As an eating plan, intermittent fasting is viable, sustainable, and a safe approach to alternative regimes to weight loss. In comparison to other eating schemes, it could not be any easier.

A fascinating study found that not only *what* you eat is important, but also *when* you eat. A biological study divided people into two groups. Over the next one hundred days, they ate the same amount and the same quality of food. One group had an early breakfast, fasted all day, and then had a late supper; the other group ate normally throughout the day. The results showed that the fasting group had a 20% weight loss and low levels of chronic inflammation, stroke, heart disease, and cancer. During all the time you eat and your body processes your food, your insulin levels are elevated due to continuous high sugar levels. Thus, your body is stuck in a fat storing mode. Only a few hours of fasting will turn fat storing into a fat burning mechanism. So, continuous nibbling and making your body store fat causes liver damage, and that can lead to obesity.

Blood sugar crashes make you feel hungry, and carbohydrates (rice, potatoes, or bread) have the highest impact on blood sugar. Not all carbohydrates are equal. Foods like soy products, beans, or grainy breads do not tend to increase the sugar spike. How many carbohydrates do you eat? For instance, eating a potato has the same impact as a tablespoon of sugar.

Can fasting make you clever? One scientific study with mice revealed that, after eating nothing but junk food, the mice started to develop learning and memory problems. Junk food made these mice fat and stupid. However, an increased protein of new nerve cells in a hippocampus grows in response to fasting, and these cells are good for memory. After switching their diet, the mice could remember where the food was and so on.

Are you already in a diabetic range? Please try your best to avoid diabetes as the possibility of having a heart attack or a stroke increases enormously. Insulin is a hormone made by the pancreas, and it helps to decrease high blood sugar levels in our body. It is also known as a fat-making hormone. On the other hand, glucagon another hormone made by the pancreas, is in charge of increasing our blood sugar levels if they fall too low.

Insulin makes you fat, high levels increase the fat stores, carbohydrates spike the levels of sugar in the blood, and this requires more and more insulin. This cycle is associated with fat deposits, cancer problems, and heart problems. Too much insulin makes you resistant to that effect, and you turn into a diabetic. Diabetes may cause impotence, blindness, or losing your limbs due to poor blood circulation.

A great habit to help you prevent diabetes is intermittent fasting. Doctors routinely recommend a healthy diet to patients with high blood glucose, but it makes a marginal difference. However, those doctors who suggested fasting, their patients' blood sugar is controlled and regulated better. This gives a chance for the insulin hormone to take a break and break the circle. This book is not a replacement of your doctor. On the contrary, please see and check with your doctor to discuss your particular case.

There are other fasting methods called *alternative fasting*, but it can be too tough physically, socially, and psychologically. It involves fasting every other day, which means one day you fast and the next day you eat as usual. It can be quite challenging, but it has powerful changes in your biochemistry, and you lose weight more quickly.

Intermittent fasting is more reasonable, realistic, and, more important, doable by eating only 500 calories two days of the week, and then five days to eat as usual. This method works better for me.

How do you fit fasting into your life? Now is the best time. Ask yourself: if not now, then when? And, once you decide when to start, make sure you fully commit to it, and you feel strong and go for it and get over it. You're on the mission now; your mission is to complete it and make it a habit. If you are tempted and think of a chocolate bar, remember again that you can eat it tomorrow when you are not fasting.

Hunger pangs are more controllable than you may think. They pass. Hunger comes in waves. Take a rumbling stomach as a good sign, a healthy message. To help you to overcome hunger pangs, go for a walk, drink plenty of water, have a hot drink, or talk to a friend—anything to make yourself busy. Don't worry, hunger will not build up and up until it becomes intolerable. It goes away.

## 5.3 - Is fasting a good or bad habit for your body?

 For me, fasting became easier every time, as my body and brain already had a memory of it, and they understood what I was going through. However, for some people who want to start fasting, they may experience side effects, as their body and brain are not used to it. Some side effects are headaches, trouble sleeping, feeling out of place, and feeling hungry. Stop if you are not feeling well or strong enough to carry on. If you find it challenging, take your time. Start it as a small habit of fasting for a few hours one day, then to six or eight hours another day, and then do twelve hours a day once or twice a week. Make it accessible and comfortable for you to do it.

Testimonies of many people say they are very pleased with their results in trying intermittent fasting. Some said that they found it mildly challenging but, thanks to it, their blood pressure came down. After a few weeks of intermittent fasting, the blood sugar levels of diabetic patients went from 7.8 mmols to 5.5 mmols.

Many people say that most diets do not work. And diet trials concluded that you lose weight for a while at the beginning of a diet. But then, they consistently produce future weight gains. Individuals lose pounds in the early months, but they return to their original weight within five years. Some they got even heavier than when they started. They found it unsustainable, not feasible, not realistic, too complicated, and too difficult to fit into their daily lives.

Intermittent fasting is easy to fit into their lives. It is tolerable and organic. They still get rewards for food, still get a life, they have a variety of food, there's no drama, no desperate diet, no self-fluctuation, and no sweat. Doctors were sceptical in the beginning to try this method, but then they started to advise their patients to try it.

Some patients reported a change in the size of their food portions. For years, they thought those portions were the ones they needed to have. Intermittent fasting is not only an eating plan; it is a lifestyle. This is a re-calibration process that will change your mind, your behaviour, and your way of life. You will cultivate an approach to eating responsibly, thoughtfully, rationally, and all without even knowing you are doing it.

Intermittent fasting feels far better than eating cakes; fasting feels good. You are no longer around food, there is no cooking, and there is no washing up. Fasters acknowledge a feeling of relief, of liberation.

Hunger is not the issue. One wonders if it suited the food industry that we developed the fear of hunger, threating us with low blood sugar and what not. Just one day of little food and you will feel emancipated, not restricted.

Before you start fasting, know your weight and body mass index (BMI). Thereafter, taking your weight once a week will suffice.

Have a target in mind, where you would like to be, and when you make a plan, write it down. It is very important that before you start intermittent fasting, make sure that you share your willingness of doing it with your doctor. Also, when you are about to start, it would be great if you could have a fasting friend, a supportive friend. Once you are on a fasting diet, tell people about it. You will not starve on your given day, and you will enjoy the food you love most of the time, just not on your two fasting days. The intermittent fasting eating plan is more manageable than any eating regime. And I feel amazing when I fast and exercise with cross trainer weights, and so on.

Let me introduce you to my colleague Wendy. We started together with the intermittent fasting (IF). While she did it mainly because she wanted to get rid of some pounds, I did it for its health benefits. The primary health benefits to fasting are: it helps with the reduction of inflammations, it reduces the risk of type 2 diabetes, it optimises the body's resistance to oxidative stress (which is related to ageing and many chronic illnesses), and, of course, it helps you to lose weight.

Wendy put on weight throughout the years, resembling her mother, and struggled with her weight most of her life. She watched her mother try different diets. Her weight remained stuck in the danger zone. Her doctor told her that she was overweight and her sort of fat was visceral fat, leading to higher risks of diabetes and cardiovascular diseases.

Thanks to intermittent fasting, Wendy dropped 20 pounds in six months. She is going to give us some tips on how she approached IF. For most of the eating regimes and weight loss programmes, the main objective is to reduce calories without malnutrition. However, compared to the other eating methods, IF is focused on when to eat.

Wendy said that intermittent fasting is not for everyone. It is not recommended for breastfeeding mothers, pregnant women, children/teenagers, underweight people, or very old people.

Make sure that before you start any fasting method, you share your interest in IF with your doctor. Wendy did not have any side effects. She did not have any sleep interruptions, and she didn't feel dizzy or about to faint at any time. If any of these side effects happen to you, stop the fasting and consult with your doctor.

I have been grateful to Wendy for her early support and guidance in adopting this life-changing lifestyle. Her journey in losing 20 pounds was what initially got me interested in researching IF. I found comfort in knowing someone who had success with it, and she felt amazing about it.

She could eat what she liked, but she didn't eat the ton of crap she used to eat. As part of this plan, she learned it was okay to feel hungry. But, in the end, it wasn't a big deal. If you feel hungry, you won't perish or feel weak, and the hunger pangs will go away.

Wendy declared that: I decided to go for the 5-2 style of fasting, and it has worked well for me too. This means I eat normally for five days during the week and fast two non-consecutive days of the week. Do I like the fact of having some days of not eating? I try to think that I do not have to bother with shopping and what to eat for lunch. I save the time of cooking, and guess what? No washing up! Apart from being very good for you, fasting is also very convenient.

I start fasting on Mondays. I take the reduction calories approach of 500 calories split over breakfast and dinnertime of that day. Let's say I had a small breakfast of around 250 calories at 07:00 a.m. and then at dinnertime I had a small dinner of around 250 calories at 07:00 p.m. The fasting time is 12 hours with some drinks in between, such as water or black herbal tea. Avoid any sweetened drinks.

The time periods can also be changed. Some of my friends prefer 09:00 a.m. and 09: 00 p.m., and so on. Choose the one that better accommodates your work/family schedule. The next day, I break my fast, and I eat my full day of meals. The total calories I eat is my TDEE (total daily energy expenditure), which is around 1800 calories. Please, you do not need to count calories, just sensibly eat your usual food patterns.

**Tips for the first two weeks of intermittent fasting**

I remember that I got better results after my first two weeks than I thought I would. Wendy also felt it a bit challenging, as her body was trying to adjust. Once we got through it, fasting became part of a habit in our lifestyle.

Here are four tips that helped me:

Let your family or friends know that you are fasting. They can be very supportive, and they may even take an interest in IF.

Have plenty of water during your fasting days.

Split your intermittent fasting into a small breakfast and supper of 250 calories each.

If, for some reason, on your fasting day you consume more than 500 calories, break your fast and eat a full day's worth of calories (your TDEE). Do not try to fast the next day and stick with your weekly schedule. Do not worry; there is always another time. Do not feel bad or guilty about it.

It is imperative to eat your full day's worth of calories since you are already eating at a deficit on your fast days. Do not try to eat less or skip meals.

After six months of your intermittent fasting, your eating habits may change, and you may find that you eat half of your meal, or you may eat more vegetables. You may find that junk food is less appealing. IF helps you to recheck your diet. You will say no to the cheesecake simply because you don't want it, and it is a long-run ticket to eliminate bad habits about food.

Your body is not my body; mine is not yours. I like beetroots, blueberries, and fennel. Whatever you eat, stick to the basic method of 500 calories of intermittent fasting. You know what fasting means. At the beginning, if you find it difficult to fast for two days in a week, make an adjustment and fast once every two weeks. Once you get used to it, you will see how your appetite will change. Expect your food preferences to adapt, and pretty soon you will start to choose healthy food by default.

Doing intermittent fasting and consuming 500 calories is a significant commitment, but as you progress, fasting will become second nature. Be smart. Spend your calories wisely. Go for a clear favourite fasting food, and implement a variety of food as well. During your intermittent fasting, bear in mind that it is more realistic and sustainable to do IF in two not-sequential days of the week.

Stick to 500 calories between breakfast and supper. You should not count calories for the rest of the days. If you feel you must eat something in between, eat carrot sticks or apples. Longer periods get better results than smaller more frequent periods. The primary aim is that you stick to the intermittent fasting for you to get the major benefits of weight loss and cheerful compliance. The key here is for you to decide and use the timetable that suits you. It is your plan and your life.

The food/calories that you should eat on your fasting days for breakfast and dinner could be cottage cheese, boiled eggs, scrambled eggs, smoked salmon, asparagus spears, tuna and beans with garlic, or haddock.  Also, cow milk cow is better than soya milk; it has a lower GI (glycaemic index) and GL (glycaemic load).

More food suggestions for your IF breakfast and dinner periods are:  go for the good proteins, steamed white fish, which are low in fat and rich in minerals, low-fat chicken, and dairy instead of endless lattes. Also, go for prawns, tuna, tofu, legumes, seeds, pulses, and nuts full of fibre. Eggs are full of nutritional value, and they will not be more than 80 calories each. They will make you feel fuller during the day than eating wheat protein. Also, fresh herbs arc virtually calorie-free.

During fasting, the amount of weight loss very much depends on how long one has been struggling with obesity; the longer the time, the harder it will be lose weight.

We need to bear in mind that intermittent fasting is no different from any other skill in life. Practise and support are paramount to doing it well, and you will learn to make it a good habit.

# Chapter 6:
# The Importance of
# Water in Our Lives

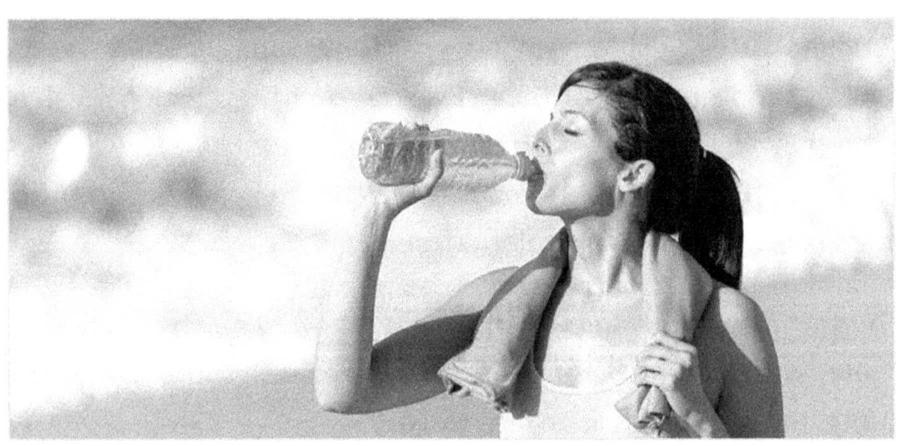

Drinking water helps you to feel amazing

# 6.1 - Why should you drink water?

I consider water as the fundamental element in our lives. Everyone is affected by this amazing element. We cannot live without it, and it is a precious, precious component in our body. Water is the odourless, tasteless, and colourless chemical substance that rules our planet and, of course, our bodies. This substance is made up of billions of molecules. Thus, each molecule consists of one oxygen and two hydrogen atoms held together by strong covalent bonds. Water is essential for life. We need water to drink, to wash, to water plants, for cooking, and many other things.

You need to keep hydrated, as it is vital for your health and well-being, and yet many people do not intake enough fluids each day. It is a vital element, and all human beings should have and enjoy it. And yet millions of people struggle to have access to clean and drinkable water.

In Westernised countries, we are so privileged that we enjoy water at any time. We don't pay much attention, and we take it for granted. But, water can also be a natural disaster. It can strike different countries in the form of hurricanes, storms, floods, tsunamis, and cyclones. It can become a disaster for many.

Nature has no pity, and it is cruel to all of us. Floods can lead to suffering, mainly in the developing countries. But not only developing nations are affected. Hurricane Katrina whipped the whole city of New Orleans in the US. After the hurricane, access to healthy water was a critical issue and a priority for survival. The thing is, we do not realise and appreciate what we have until we lose it. It's the same with water. It's a rare gold that keeps us going, and that is why it is so important to take care of it and never take it for granted.

Approximately seventy percent of the planet's surface is covered by water. While some countries experience devastating flooding, other nations suffer from aridity, which leads to an increasing problem of the shortage of water. In both cases, the affected people have to deal with the same problem, which is the lack of water for agriculture, as well as sanitary facilities, and, of course, clean drinking water.

There are around 800 million people that are having difficulties finding clean drinking water and water for sanitation facilities.

The shortage of water enormously affects a country's nutritional and agricultural situation. Without water, agriculture is not possible, and that would affect livestock farming, and that would cause a deficit in dairy produce and meat, and that would lead to famine.

Sadly, approximately 3.5 million people die every year due to the shortage of clean water and polluted drinking water. People suffer from deadly health conditions, such as diarrhoea and intestinal worms, caused by contaminated drinking water.

It is incredible that we are living on a planet surrounded by water, and yet only three and half percent of the water is fresh water made up of ice, snow, and groundwater, which is the primary source of all of our drinking water. The remaining 96.5 percent is made up of salt water.

It is estimated that in developed countries the consumption of water, including domestic use, per day is about 150 litres. However, in developing countries, such as Nigeria, it is only 16 litres per day. In these countries, millions of girls and women have to walk a long distance to get water to provide for their families, and this water is often not of drinking quality. While we are enjoying a long hot shower, others are fighting to stay alive. Let's join forces and help these people gain access to clean water.

The scale of water that we can drink varies from person to person, depending on different factors like how active they are or how much they sweat. There is no agreement on the amount of water that one has to consume daily. But health professionals suggest taking plenty of water for quenching your thirst at any time.

Others may suggest we consume up to eight glasses of fluids a day. Within this amount of our daily intake, 80% of our water comes from drinks, while the other 20% comes from the food we eat. However, how much water should you drink during exercise? For instance, studies revealed that runners who performed a high endurance exercise had a high level of water consumption that led to hyponatremia, which is low levels of sodium in the blood. This is a dangerous condition that can lead to heart failure or a heart attack and other life-threatening illnesses. Thus, overconsumption of water is not good or healthy for you either.

Our kidneys are the organs in charge of regulating our drinking water to help us to function accordingly. A kidney's function is to remove waste products and excess fluid from the body, and that it is done through the urine. The production of urine is a complex process of excretion and re-absorption, which is necessary to keep a stable balance of body chemicals—vital chemicals like salt, potassium, and acid content. Thus, if we want to perform correctly, all the cells and organs of the body need water.

Furthermore, water in our body is needed to deliver oxygen throughout the body, regulate body temperature, produce hormones and neurotransmitters, help food pass through the intestines, or cushion the brain, spinal cord, and other sensitive tissues.

Water is not only in the water itself or in beverages; there are foods with a high water content, like oranges, tomatoes, or soups.

Nephrologist researchers reported that the losses of fluids in our body occur continuously, from breathing, stools, urine, or skin evaporation; and these losses have to be replaced daily for good health. The best source of fluid for your body is by drinking water from a bottle or the tap. Drinking water instead of soda can also help with weight loss and general wellbeing.

Water also contributes to dissolving minerals and nutrients, making them more accessible to the body. It assists with removing waste products.

Your kidneys filter around 120-150 quarts on a daily basis. One quart is 1.137 litres. Of these, around 1-2 quarts are removed via the urine, and the rest is recaptured by our bloodstream. Water is a vital component for our kidney to function properly; otherwise, waste products or too many fluids could build up inside the body. A simple way to reduce the risk of kidney problems—like kidney stones and urinary tract infections—is to drink plenty of water.

Your body needs to make sure that it is hydrated all the time. If we are dehydrated, this means that we use and lose more water than we consume. Thus, this state of dehydration can lead to an imbalance in our body's electrolytes (potassium, sodium, and phosphate). Therefore, it is essential to have plenty water to facilitate proper performance of the kidneys, so they can keep the balance of electrolytes in your body. However, in severe cases of dehydration, we can be exposed to kidney failure leading to a life-threatening situation.

Let me remind you that it is not only the kidneys that are affected by a lack of water in our body. Our blood, which is 90 percent water, can get thicker without sufficient water, and that could lead to an increase in our blood pressure.

When we are in a state of dehydration, our airways are restricted, and this can make allergies or asthma conditions worse.

Dehydration may cause premature wrinkling in our skin. Moreover, our bowel requires water to function properly. A lack of water can cause digestive problems, constipation, and higher levels of acidity in the stomach, and that can contribute to the risk of heartburn and stomach ulcers. Dehydration can also affect our brain performance, as it can cause problems with thinking and reasoning.

Babies under one-year-old have a percentage of body water around 78%; then it drops to 65%. Lean tissue has more water than fatty tissue. And women have less water than men do, as a percentage.

Some medical professionals were concerned that caffeinated beverages had a diuretic effect, which means that they could cause the body to release water. However, scientific research revealed that the fluid loss is minimal.

Studies revealed that even though water has all these benefits, many people do not drink enough water, and they go for the sweetened beverages instead. Investigations revealed that approximately 40% percent of individuals drink too little water. I encourage you to start this amazing habit of drinking water accordingly, for a healthier you, and stop drinking the sweetened stuff.

## 6.2 - What are the benefits of drinking enough water?

Water is the best source of fluid in our body because it is calorie-free, alcohol-free, and caffeine-free. In spite of all the advantages and benefits water can have, it has become the second most popular drink (behind soft drinks). Water is vital on a daily basis, and it is an essential nutrient your body needs. It is present as plain water, in food, or in drinks.

It is when your water intake does not equal your output that one becomes dehydrated. Fluid loss can happen as a result of strenuous exercise, warmer climates, high altitudes, or even in older adults whose sense of thirst is not as sharp, and they do not drink as much as they should.

In our brain, there is a gland known as the pituitary. This gland communicates with your kidneys, and it is in control of how much water to excrete as urine or hold onto in reserve. When we are low in fluids, our brain triggers the body's thirst mechanism. So, if we are thirsty, a good choice is to drink water, milk, or natural juice, but not alcohol. Alcohol interferes with the brain and kidney intercommunication and produces a higher excretion of fluids, which can lead to dehydration.

Water can be an excellent contributor to help you control calories. And, substituting water for higher calorie beverages will help you for sure.

Water can also contribute to energising muscles: the cells in our body have to maintain their balance of fluids and electrolytes; otherwise, it will lead to muscle fatigue.

We need to bear in mind that when muscle cells do not have the appropriated fluids, they do not work correctly and performance can suffer. Thus it is essential to drink plenty fluids while exercising.

Water is a significant factor in keeping skin looking good. It is a fact that dehydration makes our skin look more wrinkled and dry, but your skin can get better with adequate hydration. Once we are fully hydrated, the kidneys take control and excrete excess fluids.

Water has an enormous influence on your kidneys. The role of this organ is transporting body fluids and waste products in and out of cells. A toxin, such as blood urea nitrogen, a water-soluble waste, goes through the kidney where it is excreted in the urine. Your kidney's main function is cleansing and getting rid of toxins, as long as your intake of fluids is correct. When you drink enough fluids, the urine flows freely, is light in colour, and does not have any odour. On the other hand, if you don't drink enough, the urine is concentrated, has an odour, and the colour is darker. There is a tendency to suffer from kidney stones if you chronically drink little, particularly in hot climates.

Furthermore, when there is not enough fluid in your body, the colon pulls water from stools to keep hydration, and this can lead to constipation. Thus, constipation can be diminished by intaking an adequate amount of water.

Bear in mind that the toxins in our body can activate specific natural enzymes. The function of these enzymes is to transform toxins into water-soluble substances that can be excreted from our body. The central mechanisms to help eliminate these toxins are drinking plenty of water and sweating. But, if the toxins get saturated in our fatty tissues, then the toxins can be deposited in the brain and in the body organs. As a result, over time, the contamination can accumulate and lead to various diseases. The problem with toxin residues is that they can block oxygen flow; therefore, they can inhibit the ability of nutrients to reach your individual cells. This dysfunction causes the inability to breathe and to be nourished; the cells can mutate, making themselves susceptible to illnesses and cancer.

Scientific research found that many viruses or genetic abnormalities are the ones to blame for most of these degenerative conditions. But, dehydration can be the cause of many chronic illnesses. By taking a proper amount of water, as water has natural healing properties, salts, and minerals, it can help you to prevent diseases, and even reverse the damage already done.

By drinking pure water, it can help to protect your cells from the damage of toxins. The cleansing cycle is carried on until the body is thoroughly purified and saturated with water. Get into the habit of drinking spring water, as that is the most efficient way of eliminating toxins from your body—no diet colas, or powdered drink mixes. Beverages containing artificial components are a strain on the body. Also, they may lead to dehydration and diseases, such as diabetes and hypertension.

To invert any of the illnesses produced by dehydration, it is vital to adequately supplement your body needs with intracellular minerals. Your diet must be high in magnesium, calcium, potassium, zinc, and selenium content. This is the simple solution to resolve any of the modern health conditions we have come across. Food and water can be our best medicine. Water also has some of those minerals. It is not only a source of health and well-being but as a protector against pollutants in our environment. Firstly, consuming water will diminish the damage that is caused by these pollutants, and secondly, it will immediately flush contaminants out of your body.

Stress secretes many hormones that break up new material and absorb the free water from your circulation, and that can lead to dehydration. So, every time you feel stressed, that can be due to dehydration. The primary hormones that are released when one is stressed are endorphins, vasopressin, cortisone-release-factor and prolactin, which are activated both in the kidneys and in the brain.

Many diseases are caused by dehydration. During this process, we lose a significant part of our amino acids, and they are used as antioxidants. Dehydration is also related to mineral deficiencies; due to dehydration, our body turns into an achlorhydric state (that's when the gastric secretion of the stomach and digestive organs is low or absent). This is critical, as one needs acid to absorb manganese, zinc, magnesium, selenium, and other minerals. Thus, the lack of mineral deficiency may also lead to neurological conditions such as Alzheimer's or Parkinson's disease.

Water is also a nutrient; in fact, water is the main nutrient in the body that our body depends on a regular basis for its good performance. Water has an essential role in the metabolic states of our body and regulates functions. For instance, a kilo of meat that you eat does not have energy value, unless water is there to hydrolyse it and break it down. It becomes the water that energises the food that we eat. Sugar, potatoes, and so on cannot pass energy into the human body unless water is there to break them down. Unfortunately, the water-intake-regulating mechanism of the body is not equally valid throughout the lifespan of an individual. As we get older, our perception of feeling thirst diminishes. It can happen that some elderly individuals do not recognise their thirst, and they become dehydrated more often.

To reduce hypertension problems, you need water, and you need salt to perform the reverse osmosis system. Furthermore, you need potassium, magnesium, calcium, and zinc, which are the intra-cellular minerals, to hold on to the water. Once we do this, no blood pressure will dare to increase above 120. The key is giving the body the correct amount of ingredients at the right time.

A large number of people say that salt causes the body to hold water; well this is not true. The correct ratio of water to salt will not hold water in the body. The average amount of salt that we need is approximately a gram and a half of salt to a litre of water (approx. a quarter of a teaspoon).

When we are sick in a hospital, they give us is 0.9 grams of salt per litre of water. They are not giving you the isotonic solution. Instead, they give you enough salt so your body will retain that salt.

The recommended salt to intake is sea salt, which contains around 80 trace minerals that are not in table salt. However, table salt contains iodine, which is vital, so bear in mind that sea salt does not contain iodine, which can lead to developing goitres, so have an iodine supplement such as kelp, or intake vitamin containing iodine.

Salt deficiency used to be a mode of torture. The deprivation of salt was a mechanism of a death sentence. People would die very quickly in agony without salt.

## 6.3 - What habits should you implement to help you drink plenty of water?

Here are some good habits to help you to increase your fluid intake and receive the benefits of water.

Habit one: Get used to having water with every meal.

Habit two: Choose beverages you enjoy, but if you are watching your figure, go for non-caloric drinks or water.

Habit three: Eat more vegetables and fruits. They have a high water content, which helps you with your hydration. Twenty percent of our fluid intake comes from foods.

Habit four: Adopt the habit of carrying a bottle of water with you at all times, in your bag, in your car, in your desk, etc.

For me, drinking water has been a habit since I was little. I was always amazed at how our body works, and how our cells needed water for our survival and healthy wellbeing. I drink plenty of water. In fact, water is the main drink that I consume.

As I mentioned earlier, water is essential to keep your body healthy and active. A high percentage of our body is made of water; approximately two-thirds of an adult is composed of salt water. Although we drink fresh water, we are saline. The main reason we need to drink so much water is to keep our body's salt concentrations low, which helps to ease stress on our kidneys and cardiovascular pathways. The amount of water that is eliminated from our body is approximately eight glasses of water a day, by crying, salivating, and urinating. That is why it is so important to replace what is lost.

The way we perceive thirst is by feeling tired when we have not done a good day's work. In the morning when you wake up, if you do not feel like getting out of the bed, you are dehydrated, as you haven't had a drink for six to eight hours, depending on how many hours you sleep. Therefore, it is very important to drink water straight away. We have deprived our brain of energy; if we are dehydrated, we have a specific tendency of feeling tired. Water is our pick-me-up. Some thirst signals of the human body are asthma, allergies, hypertension, old age, diabetes, and auto-immune diseases.

You can keep healthy by drinking water accordingly. A good reminder to ourselves to prevent dehydration is that first you need water and salt on a regular basis. Also, one needs daily exercise, as our brain chemistry depends on how we move our muscles. When we exercise, we move our muscles, and then we burn the amino-acids chain, which are participants in tryptophan passage through the blood-brain barrier. It is when we burn the amino acids that our body chemistry will begin to function normally. The muscles of our calves are like our secondary hearts for venous circulation. That is why we need to exercise every day.

As a habit, I usually drink one or two glasses of water as soon as I wake up, as I know the importance of getting hydrated straight away, after a whole night's sleep. Also, every time I plan to eat, I drink water half an hour before my food. As a rule of thumb, if we expect to digest food, it is better to drink water beforehand. And I make sure that I drink plenty of water throughout the day.

Another benefit of a good habit of drinking water is that it helps to maintain normal bowel functions. A hydrated gastrointestinal tract helps to maintain a normal bowel function and helps prevent constipation. Your bowel needs adequate fluids and fibre intake, as the fluids pump up the fibre and act like a broom, which helps to keep your bowel functioning properly.

This tip is to keep you young: the more we keep our body hydrated with water, the fewer wrinkles and the effects of ageing may occur. Simplify your life by taking plenty of pure water on a daily basis. Water has an immense supporting role that it plays in biochemical processes by influencing the shape of molecules. Water, the life-sustaining solvent, regulates the functions of all systems.

Meet my friend Monica. She used to suffer from headaches. Studies revealed that dehydration could lead to the brain shrinking and that could produce headaches. She works in the community as a nurse. Monica has a family to look after and a very demanding job. She is a busy soul, looking after a family and provide care for her patients in the community.

She is so busy with her life that she sometimes forgets to drink enough water. She knows that, but with the rushes of her own life and then at work, she forgets to make sure she drinks plenty and eats well. Even though she has no significant problems with her health, her eating patterns are not that great. She is so busy and feels so tired when she finishes her shift, that she has no time or willingness to cook. So, she spoiled her palate by eating the wrong stuff, especially, processed food and processed juices.

One day, she told me that sometimes she forgets to drink enough, and she has persistent headaches. I told her that it could be because she was dehydrated by not drinking enough water. I emphasised WATER to her, not processed juices. So, she decided to drink more water, anything to get rid of the headaches. Well, guess what? Yes, her headaches disappeared once she made sure that she was drinking plenty throughout the day.

As a health practitioner, I always recommend and encourage my patients to drink plenty of fluids and water in particular. We are all exposed to environmental toxins like colds and coughs. Water is the most effective of all fluids to help get rid of all those toxins.

I make this habit of taking a bottle of water wherever I go, so what are you waiting for? Not only will you feel better, but you'll also flush out toxins quickly, and you'll feel amazing and more energetic.

A good tip to bring your weight down is by preloading meals with water. By following this habit, it can help you to shave hundreds of calories from your daily intake. Research showed that by having two cups of water just before eating, people consumed around 90 calories less over the course of a meal.

Also, bear in mind that if you feel like having a snack, think twice and first try a glass of water and then wait for ten or fifteen minutes to see if the hunger or craving has gone.

Water is a blessing. Only by realising, understanding, and honouring the true nature of water will humankind achieve a world free of disease and pollution. Give the gift of water; give the gift of life.

# Chapter 7:
# What Are Superfoods?

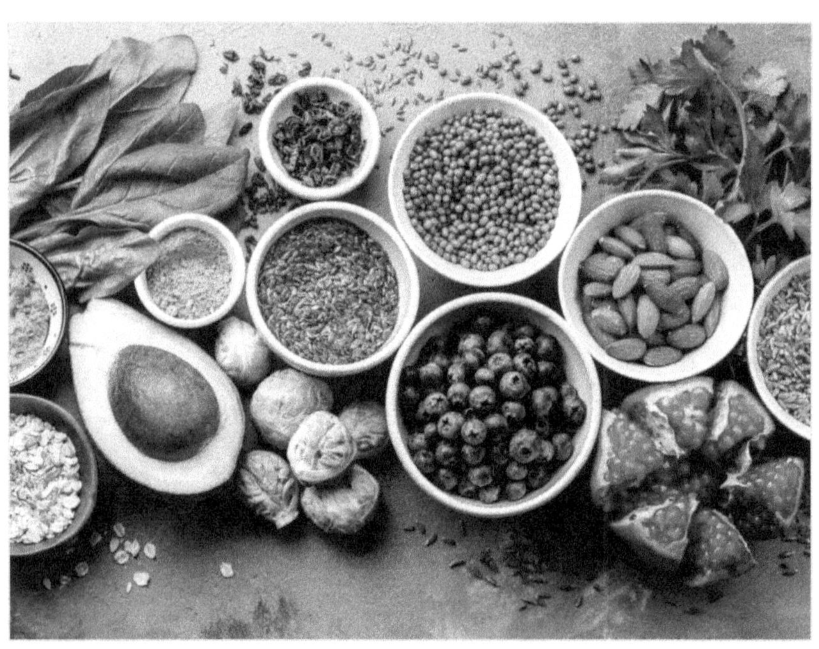

Superfoods have great benefits for your health

# 7.1 - What are superfoods, and is it advisable to eat them?

The so-called 'superfoods' have become more popular than ever due to their high nutritional content and different health benefits. The nutrition experts define superfood as low-calorie and containing high levels of minerals, vitamins, antioxidants, and polyphenols (the specific element that helps to protect radicals).

Thus, superfoods are also known to fight free radicals, a kind of oxygen molecule that is considered to be a component in causing some illnesses, among them are cancer, diabetes, and the ageing process. Blueberries have a high level of antioxidants, which aim to preserve against these free radicals. Blueberries help with memory problems as well.

You should include superfoods as part of your diet, as they can help you to lose weight, boost your energy levels, improve your skin and hair, and minimise the risk of digestive problems and chronic diseases.

The British Dietetic Association revealed that a high percentage of people (up to 61%) stated that they had bought a particular food or drink just because it was labelled as a superfood.

Superfoods can be plant-based like kale or acai, but they can also be found in some fish (salmon) and dairy, as these products are nutritionally dense and thus good for your health.

So, what does *superfoods* mean? This term is not scientific. The term has led to plenty of debates over the fact that some consumers will eat one type of food over another if it is labelled as a superfood. Is broccoli superior to asparagus?

The key elements in an ideal diet are those that contain a wide variety of vegetables, fruits, healthy animal products, and whole grains.

There is no doubt that superfoods might be a good entry into healthy eating, and understanding the nutritional value of the food you eat can be enlightening. But, do not be misled, as there are lots of healthy foods out there to explore, even if no one is calling them 'super' food.

Furthermore, the so-called superfoods and the health claims have been banned by the European Union on packaging unless supported by scientific evidence.

Therefore, there are no specific criteria to determine which foods are *super*foods. Dieticians believe that 'superfood' is a marketing term for foods that contain health benefits.

The idea of consuming so-called superfoods that are packed with nutrients is undoubtedly a good idea. To eat healthily, you need balanced and nutritious foods within the right quantities.

There are popular, and therefore favourite, superfoods preferred by the public. This kind of food tends to have extra-large doses of minerals and vitamins that can contribute to ward off diseases and help a person live a longer and healthier life. Superfoods contain healthy fats, fibres, and antioxidants.

One of the top superfoods I have chosen to eat is blueberries, as they contain plenty of soluble fibre, and they are rich in vitamins. But, the same kind of nutrients that are found in blueberries can be found in other types of berries, like cranberries or strawberries.

Also, one of my favourite superfoods is kiwi fruit. This fruit has similar benefits to melons, apples, or citrus fruit, which all contain a high level of vitamin C, and they are rich in antioxidants. Moreover, the kiwi fruit is identified as a superfood because of its more extensive range of nutrients in comparison to other fruits. Kiwifruit also contains serotonin, which is a hormone that helps regulate and maintain sleep. Thus, it might help to promote a better night's rest in people with sleeping problems.

Beans and whole grains, which form part of the qualified superfoods lists, are a source of low-fat protein. And, beans provide insoluble fibre, which helps to lower your cholesterol. Also, beans give you a more prolonged feeling of fullness.

Whole grains are known by this name, as, unlike refined grains, they are not stripped of their nutrient-containing bran and germ during processing. Quinoa is not considered as a grain, but it cooks up like one. It is an excellent source of vitamins, proteins, minerals, antioxidants, and fibre.

However, it is important to cite that many whole grains are processed for a better delicious taste, and they are less healthful. For instance, and unfortunately, in the markets, we see more and more instant whole-grain oats. This means that they are processed food, and therefore they are considered to be as unhealthy as overly processed white bread. Once those oats are consumed, one of the unhealthy effects is that they quickly spike the sugar levels in the bloodstream, which can contribute to insulin resistance, diabetes, or obesity.

## 7.2 - What are the benefits of eating superfoods?

Dieticians certainly encourage their clients to eat everything in moderation. Dieticians want you to keep in mind that those foods labelled as 'superfoods' have the properties of being 'super' and 'healthy,' but be careful of the quantity you consume. Just because they are healthy, you can't eat as much as you'd like. As in everything in life, moderation is the key to a functional and wellbeing status. So, you have to be cautious of the quantity you consume, as you can gain weight from overeating healthy foods too.

Now, more than ever, people tend to have the latest and best lifestyle choices, and this includes our daily eating and how we can reduce our risk of chronic diseases like cancer, stroke, or heart conditions. Thus, the food industry wants to take part and convince us that eating a specific food, a 'super' food, can slow down the ageing process, boost our physical abilities, and lift depression.

Many of us want to believe that eating a single fruit or vegetable containing a certain antioxidant will zap a diseased cell, and that would not be great!

All unprocessed food from the major food groups (proteins, fat, or carbohydrates) could be considered 'super.' All these foods are valuable as part of a balanced diet.

Dieticians avoid the term 'superfood' and prefer to talk about a super eating plan, where the emphasis is on healthy, good, and nutritious eating, rich in fruits and vegetables and wholegrains foods.

Studies revealed that the Mediterranean way of eating is good evidence that it can reduce the risk of some chronic health conditions, and it can increase life expectancy. This diet contains plenty of vegetables, legumes, olive oil, and fruit, and less meat and dairy foods than the typical Western diet.

You should eat in moderation a variety of foods to ensure that you get enough of the nutrients your body needs. It is so essential that our health and diet should not concentrate on individual foods, as that may encourage unhealthy eating. You need to be clear that not any superfood food can compensate for your unhealthy eating. And do not mistakenly think that superfoods can undo the damage produced by unhealthy foods. For you to eat well is about consuming healthy foods at all times.

Be cautious with superfoods, as it seems they are trending. Kale is one of them now. Spinach was prior, and the next one is turmeric spice.

So, what if you cannot afford to buy these fancy superfoods, or they are not available, or you cannot afford to pay for some of the pricier superfoods?

There are no standard criteria for the approved list of superfoods. Dieticians recommend getting your nutritional benefits by eating any variety of vegetables, fruits, yoghurts, and walnuts. Antioxidant-rich foods include a variety of berries, peppers, and anything rich in vitamin C, like papaya, grapefruits, and oranges, or rich in vitamin A, such as carrots. What I would also like to see people eat more of are the superfoods like whole grains, legumes, nuts and seeds, fish, and all fruits and vegetables.

'Practically everything in the produce department is a superfood.'

Yoghurt is very nutritious and widely available. It could also be considered as a superfood. It contains a high source of calcium, protein, and fat. One tip to add to have an excellent mini-meal is to add fruit or walnuts to your yoghurt. It is about to encourage you to start with the basics and then to move their way upwards. When you eat all these superfoods, you do not have to take a multivitamin. Thus, by intaking superfoods, they can help you to get a more authentic and healthy form of nutrients into your body, rather than just popping a multivitamin.

The best thing reported about superfoods is their high levels of antioxidants. But dieticians report that all vegetables and fruits have antioxidants. They recommend eating a wide variety of fruits and vegetables each day, in particular, brightly coloured ones like strawberries or dark leafy greens such as spinach.

You may feel bombarded about superfoods, how they can be a passing fad diet, or ads touting their health benefits. Superfoods claim everything from promoting weight loss to slowing ageing. The glut of information can be overwhelming.

So, do superfoods reduce the risk of heart disease and stroke?

Studies have found that superfoods are good for your heart and your overall health. The incorporation of superfoods has to be balanced in fruits, whole grains, vegetables, low-fat milk, dairy products, and lean proteins, in addition to legumes, fish, nuts, and seeds.

But are they really 'super'?

Marketing efforts perpetuate most myths about superfoods.

A lot of people have unrealistic expectations about these foods, thinking they will be protected from chronic diseases and health problems. They may add one or two of these superfoods on the top of their poor diet, but this will not help or protect anything. The U.S. Department of Agriculture reported that many people have very poor eating patterns. And there are still many individuals that do not intake enough calcium, vitamin D, potassium, and dietary fibre, which are all found easily in whole grains, milk, vegetables, and fruits.

One of the best superfoods is avocado. They have some properties that help the fight against wrinkles, due to the high level of antioxidants, as well vitamins, potassium, and good fats.

Avocados are good for a longer life. They are considered as superfood thanks to their potent compounds that can also help to regenerate the cells of your body. Among these compounds, there is one called xanthophyll, which is a powerful antioxidant. Scientific studies reported that an intake of xanthophyll is likely to contribute to reducing signs of ageing on different parts of the body. Also, avocados are good for wound healing, and they can help repair dry, damaged, or chapped skin. And, when it comes to taste, avocados are a very soft food where you combine different foods and ingredients to find your ideal and tasty recipe.

Legumes, such as lentils, soybeans, and chickpeas, have anti-ageing properties, and they are low in fat. They are also a good source of vegetable protein fibre. They are good for cholesterol, joints, and blood pressure, and they can also improve your digestive health.

Good news for chocolate lovers—nutrition experts revealed that dark chocolate, yes it has to be dark chocolate, is useful to protect the body from cancer and heart conditions due to the high level of antioxidants and polyphenols. But, remember to eat chocolate with moderation!

Oats help to improve your skin. They are also suitable if you are stressed or tired. Porridge or oats contain vitamin E, potassium, calcium, protein, and magnesium.

Watercress is a delicious and simple food. They are straightforward to use as a salad accessory or sandwich ingredient. They contain vitamins A and C.

Chia seeds are full of antioxidants and omega 3. Just one tablespoon of chia seeds has more calcium than a cup of milk.

Spirulina is a freshwater alga, often known as the original superfood. It contains all the essential amino acids and proteins, and it is an excellent detoxifier.

Some superfoods are known to aid digestion, fight heart disease, protect organs from toxins, reduce inflammation in the body, regulate metabolism, lower cholesterol, and fight cancer.

While many food product marketers are jumping on the superfood bandwagon, stay focused on selecting unprocessed, natural foods for maximum benefits. And, of course, it is essential to include a broad range of foods types in your diet. They work better together, so add a variety of fresh fruits, veggies, and whole grains for a balanced diet and optimal health. Among them: oily fish, berries, tomatoes, broccoli, linseeds, natural yoghurt, tea, ginger, soy.

Researchers found that eating more brightly coloured fruits and vegetables is a simple way to improve your health dramatically.

Researchers have found that by eating seven or more portions of vegetables and fruits daily, it decreases the risk of death from any cause, at any point in time, by a whopping 42%!

Despite these staggering statistics, the unfortunate truth is that very few people manage to achieve anything near this. A survey showed that only 31% of adults aged 19 to 64 and 37% aged 65 and over are making the bare minimum recommendations of at least five portions daily. We now know that it's seven or even nine portions a day that will provide more significant benefits.

A lot of has been written about the benefits of an alkaline diet. Eating more fresh vegetables and fruits promotes a more alkaline pH, which, in part, can positively influence many aspects of your health, such as your levels of energy, immune balance, cancer risk, diabetes risk, and blood sugar balance. Moreover, by eating more vegetables and fruits, you have also increased your intake of minerals, such as zinc, magnesium, and potassium.

It is a said that calcium intake helps you to strengthen your bones, and calcium is found in dairy products. Not many people are aware of the properties of veggies and fruits and their significant impact on bone health too. Vegetables and fruits promote an alkaline pH, which is the right component to build healthy bones. On the other hand, when the pH is more acidic, where a typical Western diet can find it, calcium must be released from the bones to bring the pH back into balance. These imbalances in the bones weaken them leading to the risk of osteoporosis. Thus, it is essential to have a diet rich in vegetables and fruits to build healthy bones and decrease the risk of osteoporosis.

## 7.3 - What habits should you follow concerning superfoods?

You can boost your energy, drop pounds, and feel amazing with these eating plan adjustments.

You should have a plan for having a balanced diet throughout the day. For instance, if you are planning to go out for a steak and potatoes at lunch, go easy on the meat and starches at dinner. You should also ensure that you fit in healthy eating like whole grains, veggies, nuts, and fruits in the other meals in that day.

This forms part of having a balanced diet, and means you can ditch the habit of counting calories. But, you should get into the habit of focusing on foods that are good for you and your metabolism. Instead of asking how many calories, ask yourself where the food came from and if it is it nutritious.

I know from experience that eating healthy, nutrient-rich foods keeps my hunger at bay, helps me to maintain stable blood sugar levels, and minimises my cravings.

A good habit of eating healthy and balanced meals is eating more vegetables. So, cook your veggies in a way that saves the high flavour. And lose the way of thinking that 'healthy' equals 'tasteless.' Thus, your vegetables can be a delicious meal and not boring, and there are thousands of recipes for vegetables!

Get into the habit of spending time on food preparation, as it is linked to better eating habits. We are creatures of habits, and, therefore, it is all about convenience. One tip, for instance, is when you get home from the shop or supermarkets with the bounty of fruits and veggies in tow, wash and chop them right away and store them in a container in your fridge. If they are ready for you, you will grab them in a pinch. If not? It is chips and dips time, right? You can do the same with other foods, like making roasting a bunch of veggies to throw together for quick lunches.

Eat the rainbow—get into the habit of eating a variety of veggies and fruits, as they will supply your body with a range of illness-fighting phytonutrients. At the same time, they will fill you up and help you cut back on unhealthy foods. Studies revealed that a variety of vegetables encourage you to eat more of them, so make your plate a rainbow of food!

If you are not willing to change or give up your snacks, ensure you eat healthy snacks. After all, the high percentage of snacking is one of the reasons for the rise in calorie intake over the last few decades. Snacking habits are adding too many calories and too few nutrients to our diets. When done right, snacking keeps your energy levels up and gives you more opportunities to get all your nutritional needs. This means that your fridge or desk should be stocked with an emergency stash of snacks, like individual packs of nuts, dried fruit, Greek yoghurt, or go for picking a protein-fruit pairing of a cup of skim milk and an apple.

Minty iced green tea is a calorie-free beverage that does not qualify as a real snack. But, if you find yourself searching the kitchen just because you're bored, rather than hungry, this tasty drink may just hit the spot. Also, studies showed that green tea has some properties to help you lose weight thanks to its metabolism-boosting antioxidant compound known EGCG.

Asparagus and hard-boiled egg: this combination goes so well, as the fibre-rich asparagus balances out the eggs' natural protein.

Lentil salad with tomatoes and watercress: salads are not just for mealtimes. As they are low in calories, they can be part of a fantastic afternoon snack, as well. This one has 11 grams of protein and 8 grams of fibre, thanks to superfood lentils and plenty of veggies.

I would like to share with you my own experience about avoiding snacks. As I mentioned earlier, I work as a nurse. I am in the habit of having three meals per day, fasting, and avoiding snacks, and it works perfectly fine for me. My colleagues are amused about my integrity with food, as I do not snack. They are surprised that I didn't eat any snacks, while they can't stop snacking. They asked me about it, and I explained to them the importance of setting up proper habits with regard to the food that one eats. I keep telling them that the best medicine that one can have is good and nutritious food if one wants to be free of abdominal pains, digestive discomforts, and so on. That is why your mind-set is so important. I don't remember being sick or unwell even once. I don't have any days where I don't go to work because I feel sick.

I wanted to encourage my colleagues to change their mind-set and habits associated with their eating patterns. I wanted them to realise that having abdominal discomforts after eating a heavy meal, or that constant cravings and wanting to snack all the time when they don't even feel hungry is not natural. I kept telling them our body does not need to eat many times during the day. In fact, our body needs to have a break from eating.

The foods that we eat are all foods that make us feel good or bad. So many processed foods, with so many different additives and preservatives, cannot be suitable for our body! Eating processed foods full of sugar or simple carbohydrates that make your insulin work harder can lead to insulin resistance. This means an increase in your sugar levels, and, therefore, more fat in your body leading to obesity. We need to put into our frame of mind how vital it is to eat well, so it will help us to feel amazing.

# Chapter 8:
# Exercise

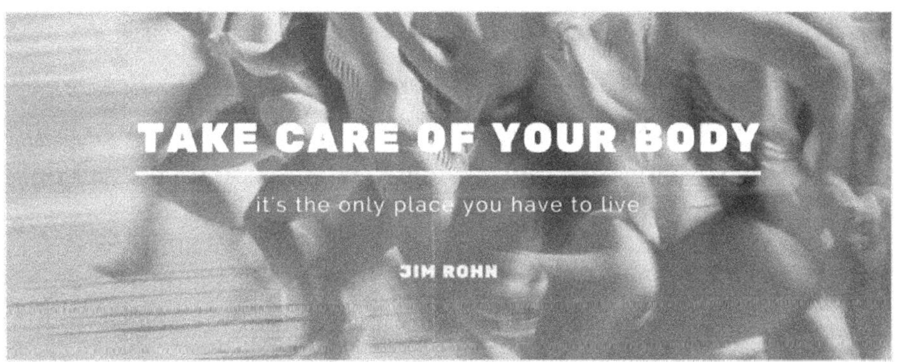


## 8.1 - Does exercise help you to lose weight?

There are a lot of debates about the value of doing exercise and losing weight. While there are plenty of studies, experts who study exercise—and the thousands of individuals who have lost weight—all corroborate that working out works.

The following will explain valuable information about what happens in our body when we exercise.

Studies have shown that regular aerobic exercise is the best way to lose weight; it has the most significant impact on decreasing abdominal fat. This kind of fat is a danger to your health, as it can lead to the risk of diabetes or a heart condition. Also, exercise helps to lower levels of cortisol, which is a hormone associated with abdominal fat. In fact, studies revealed that women with a higher percentage of cortisol in their system have a more prominent body mass index and bellies than those with lower amounts of this hormone.

Of course, you will lose fat when you diet without exercising, but exercising also affects your muscles too. Once you build your muscles, your metabolism will be higher, and you will burn more calories. In fact, when you burn fat and gain muscle, you may lose inches and fall in sizes without actually losing any pounds. Thus, if you gained four pounds of lean muscle, and lost five pounds of fat, you have improved nine pounds in your body shape; despite the scale only showing one pound of weight loss.

It's a straightforward thing—regular exercise burns excess calories that would otherwise be stored as fat.

However, research has shown that exercise will not contribute to you losing weight nearly as much as most people think.

People expect that exercising will help them to lose all the weight they want to lose.

There are different theories about losing weight. Some doctors claim that exercise is right for you, but it will not help you to lose weight. There is a contradiction among studies indicating that working out increases your base metabolic rate, meaning you burn more calories throughout the day. The critical factor is that if you exercised for over three months with no intention of changing your diet, you would only lose 1 pound. Obviously, we know that exercise is essential for our health, but studies reveal that exercise alone will not cause enough weight loss. And diet is the primary focus of weight loss.

Researchers challenge obesity-prevention strategies that exercise alone is not enough to lose weight for the same reason our bodies reach a plateau where working out more does not necessarily burn extra calories.

Let me introduce my good friend Java. She is one of the people who always believed that if she worked out hard, she would get the reward. At the end of a sixty-minute workout, her body was dripping with sweat. She felt like she had worked hard. And according to her bike, she had burned more than 700 calories. Surely, she had earned an extra milkshake!

Exercise, of course, is one of the ways of making us hungry. Studies have shown that individuals seemed to increase their food intake after exercise, either because they thought they burned a significant amount of calories or because they felt hungrier after they worked out.

One works hard, working out tremendously for an hour, and that hard work can be erased with a few minutes of bad eating afterwards.

For instance, one slice of pizza could undo the calories burned off in a sixty-minute workout. Furthermore, after a workout, people simply slow down, and they burn less energy on their non-gym exercises; for instance, they will take a lift instead of using the stairs. This way of acting is known as compensatory behaviours, and they are associated with adjustments one may unconsciously make after working out to counteract the calories burned.

Countless studies have demonstrated that exercise contributes in a modest way in losing weight, meaning that it helps us maintain our weight.

Those studies showed that exercise is entirely unhelpful for weight loss. Our energy comes 100% from our food intake. We can only burn approximately 10% to 30% of it with physical activity each day.

One has to be mindful, and you should not expect to be able to lose a lot of weight by ramping up your physical activity. While exercise is vital for our general health, the critical point here is how much and what one eats has a much more significant impact on your waistline.

There is a huge problem with the obesity epidemic. Poor exercise activity and eating too many sugars and starches are equally responsible for it. Public Health departments must prioritise fighting over-consumption of low-quality food and improving the food environment.

Another research group studied a hunter tribe known as the Hadza (who were not obese). Researchers thought that they would find evidence about why obesity has become a huge problem worldwide. Many argued that one of the reasons for gaining weight over the past fifty years is that we exercise less than our ancestors did.

During this study, the researchers revealed that the energy expenditure among the Hadza was not greater than it is for people in the Westernised countries. It was an astonishing result. While the hunters were much more active, they burned the same amount of calories every day as the average European.

This study created the question: how could the Hadza hunters possibly burn the same amount of energy as indolent Europeans?

The scientists have revealed that energy expenditure, or calories burned each day, involves not only movement but all the energy required to carry out the over one hundred functions that keep us alive, like breathing, and so on.

Calorie burning has become a trait humans have evolved and it doesn't have much to do with lifestyle. The hunter tribe's researchers thought that this tribe was using the same amount of energy as Europeans, because their bodies were conserving energy on other tasks. Or perhaps the Hadza hunters were resting more when they weren't hunting to make up for all their physical activity, which would also decrease the general energy expenditure.

This science is still evolving. But it has revealed deep implications for how we think about how profoundly hardwired energy expenditure is and the scale to which we can hack it with more exercise.

If the calories out variable cannot be managed that well, what might be responsible then for the difference in the Hadza's weights?

The Hadza tribe are burning the same energy, but they do not suffer from obesity as Westerners do. The researchers claim that the hunters do not overeat; therefore, they do not become obese.

On the other hand, further studies done on exercising revealed a modest weight loss could be contributed to exercise for somebody who follows a regime. On the contrary, exercise does have a great impact on your body and your mind. There are benefits like decreasing the risk of type 2 diabetes, heart attack, and stroke, and bringing down a high cholesterol level or high blood pressure level.

The benefit of exercise is a real wonder. Some studies have found that there is very little correlation between the amount of exercise and its energy expenditure with weight loss.

Other studies had a closer look in exploring the effects of more exercise on weight, from people who trained for marathons to sedentary counters and post-menopausal overweight and obese women who did exercise such as running, or personal training sessions, or cycling. During these studies, the vast majority of these people usually only lost a few pounds at best. Thus, the conclusion of the evidence from these studies on exercise for weight loss revealed that exercise alone led to only modest reductions.

Throughout all these years, we thought of weight loss in simple calories in, calories out terms. Max Wishnofsky, a researcher in the 1950s, outlined a rule that many organisations (Livestrong to Mayo Clinic) use to predict weight loss. A pound of human fat represents about 3,500 calories; thus, burning 500 calories per day, through diet or exercise, ends up in about a pound of weight loss per week.

Nowadays, researchers see this rule as remarkably simplistic. Now, they see the human energy balance as a dynamic and adaptable system. When one alters one element, like reducing the number of calories one eats in a day or doing more physical activity than usual, this leads to a cascade of changes in the body that influence how many calories one uses up, and in turn, one's body weight.

The main elements of energy expenditure are the basal metabolic rate or the amount of energy required for performance when the body is at rest, the energy needed to break down food, and the power required during exercise or physical activity.

We have hardly any control over our basal metabolic rate, but it is our most significant energy domain. It uses approximately 60% to 80% of our overall energy expenditure, and that leaves exercise as  only a subset.

More and more evidence has been shown that exercise is not that relevant for weight loss, while it is very good for your health. Scientists have found a phenomenon called metabolic compensation associated with our physical activity work out. Physiologists think there are changes in our physiologically-compensatory mechanisms that change and reach a limit in relation to the amount of exercise we do. Therefore, it appears that our bodies may actively fight our efforts to lose weight.

A study published in 2016 looked at fourteen participants of the Biggest Loser reality TV show. Measurements were taken: hormones, fat, body weight, and metabolism. The researchers checked the contestants at the end of the show and then six years later.

The results were astonishing. Even though all the contestants lost kilos through extreme diets and hours of physical activity at the end of the show, by the time six years had passed, their waistlines had mostly rebounded. The most relevant finding was the contestants' metabolism had hugely slowed down through the study period. They were burning approximately 500 calories fewer per day than would be expected given their weight.

This metabolic element continued, in spite of the fact that most contestants were slowly regaining the weight they lost.

This factor or phenomenon is part of our survival mechanism. Our body has the ability to conserve energy and hold on to stored fat for future energy requirements.

Another theory about why our bodies are resistant to losing weight through physical activity alone is that energy expenditure reaches a state of little or no change after a period of activity at a certain point.

One study involved participants from different countries and cultures in Africa and the United States. They gathered data by using accelerometers on physical activity and energy burned. They sub-divided the participants into three types: the super active (people who exercised on a daily basis), the moderately active (people who exercised about three times a week), and the sedentary type.

The results were that the physical activity accounted for approximately eight percent of the variation in calories burned among the groups.

The researchers in the study concluded that total energy expenditure seems to be correlated with exercise, but the relationship was more prominent over the lower range of the physical activity. Thus, after a certain amount of physical activity, one does not keep burning calories at the same level: total energy expenditure may plateau after a period of time.

Researchers recalled that the energy expenditure that it shows on the effect of more physical activity on the human being is not linear.

So, it is vital to exercise just for the health improvement and not for the sake of weight loss. Dieticians and food experts on weight loss recommend stick to limited number of calories that you can sustain, and the main thing is to eat healthfully.

Losing weight is quite a complex process; there are different factors to consider. If an individual wanted to lose weight, they should do 60 minutes of average exercise (running) four times per week, while keeping his/her standard calorie intake the same. He/she would then lose about five pounds per month. Moreover, if this individual decided to raise their food consumption or relax more to recover from the added exercise, then the weight loss would be less. Therefore, if one is obese or overweight, and willing to lose kilos, it would take a significant amount of time, effort, and willingness to make a real impact through exercise.

## 8.2 - How does exercise benefit your health?

An exercise that can help you to achieve that mental and physical well-being status is fast-paced running. You can't go wrong with running. It's free and very simple to do. Follow your rhythm; do not follow the masses. Like everything in life, everything is relative. What one person may consider a fast-paced run is very different from what another person may think. Act according to your comfort, and don't try to kill yourself chasing somebody else who may have a faster pace than yours. Follow your own pace. Remember, you are not in a competition!

Running is one of the purest exercises you can do because it doesn't require any equipment.

According to dieticians and nutritionists, the best way to implement this exercise is to take 10-20 second sprints and then jog or walk for around 60 seconds. You should take the initiative of starting this new habit, and it should be repeated until you get tired.

When you exercise, it kind of creates a healthy chain of habits. In general, people tend to work on another health improvement thing, such as eating healthier. It is an added value to do exercise that can be fun. And, individuals who diet and do physical activity at the same time tend to be less hungry than those who only diet. Exercise will increase your energy, as regular exercise raises your stamina by elevating your body's production of energy-promoting neurotransmitters.

Jumping a rope is quite fun. I still remember jumping a rope during playground break at school. While thinking of school while jumping rope, I could carry on and on. It is so wonderful to be a child. Throughout the years, one realises that jumping a rope is one of the best exercises one can do to speed up our heart rate. For many boxers like Muhammad Ali, jumping rope is a way to train their footwork.

Just a few minutes of jumping rope and one notices very quickly how it can get our lungs burning and our heart racing. Now, the challenge is being able to continue it for over a few minutes non-stop.

One good habit is to jump rope in intervals. Jump rope for a specified number of reps, say 90; then walk around for 50 seconds. Then repeat this until you're too tired to jump any more.

To maximize your results, make yourself keep exercising for several minutes before you stop. Otherwise, follow the interval approach to optimise your results. During my childhood, I could jump the rope forever, but for now, I think I'll stick to the interval approach.

It's also a good idea to add swimming to your exercise habit.

The beneficial aspect of swimming is just for the single reason of being in the water; your body will burn calories while you're in the water. Our body runs typically at 98 degrees, but the average pool temperature is approximately 80 degrees. Thus, our body burns calories just by trying to keep warm and make up for the near 20-degree difference. The main benefits of swimming are for your heart and lungs, endurance and muscle strength, and to help you maintain your weight.

Of the leading martial arts, taekwondo (or Tae Kwon Do) is considered the one that burns the most calories. Its origin dates back 2,000 years in Korea. This martial art emphasises concentration, speed, power, breath control, and reaction force.

Tennis: One of the challenges of playing tennis is the rapid deceleration and acceleration, and that is the benefit of playing tennis to get fit.

Exercise is vital for your health. That is the main message we need to give to the public. There are plenty of studies that found that exercise is great for keeping our minds and bodies healthy.

The main highlights of doing exercise are the reduced risk of a range of illnesses, such as coronary heart condition, stroke, type 2 diabetes, and a variety of cancers.

Other evidence claims that the most effective way of losing weight is to minimise your refined carbohydrates intake through a healthily balanced diet habit.

Cardiologists advised the National Obesity Forum We know exercising in the right way has many health benefits, but weight loss is not one of them. We need to disassociate obesity with exercise altogether. If we're going to combat obesity, it is going to happen purely from changing the food environment.

Statistics show that one in four adults in England gets less than 30 minutes of exercise a week, and only about one-quarter of the adults eat the recommended five portions of vegetables and fruit per day.

The Public Health England department encouraged the public to be more physically active. The key to a good habit is that just by doing a little, it often makes a huge difference. Only ten minutes of extra walking per day can improve your health and your overall quality of life.

Cardiologists also encourage the public to be more active with a good reminder that being inactive can hugely increase one's risk of having a stroke or a deadly heart attack.

Okay, no need to despair. The good news is that it is never too late to start doing exercise and being more active. Being active helps reduce your cholesterol and high blood pressure, and it also improves your mental health.

The recommendation for physical activity on a weekly basis is two and a half hours. This may be a lot, but a good habit that one can follow is to break it down into ten-minute sessions per day and gradually build it up.

Studies have also revealed that exercise decreased the risk of developing cognitive impairments like dementia or Alzheimer's.

If you are trying to lose weight, exercise would be part of weight maintenance along with watching sugary and simple carbohydrate food intake. Get into this habit. Researchers have found some things in common with people who have had success losing weight. They weigh themselves at least once a week. They restrict their calorie intake, stay away from high-carb foods, and watch their portion sizes. They also exercise on a regular basis.

It seems we are in a continuing battle. The myth of physical activity is still usually deployed by the food and beverage industry, which are continuously in a hot spot for selling us so many unhealthy products. Remember, just because a product is out there, that doesn't mean that it is good for your body or your health. Stick to the healthy food and drink products.

There is plenty of evidence that exercise can help us lead a healthier and a happier life. Exercise can be considered as the miracle cure we have always had, and, yet, people neglect to exercise. If that's the case, their health could suffer as a consequence.

Researchers reveal that exercise can help you to reduce the risk of many chronic conditions, such as stroke, some cancers, type 2 diabetes, and heart disease. Moreover, physical activity can also boost your mood, energy, and self-esteem, as well minimising the risks of stress, dementia, and depression.

Dr Nick Cavill, who is a health promotion consultant, said, If exercise were a pill, it would be one of the most cost-effective drugs ever invented.

It has been proven through research that people who regularly exercise have:

- a 30% lower risk of early death

- a 20% lower risk of breast cancer

- an 83% lower risk of osteoarthritis

- a 68% lower risk of hip fracture

- a 30% lower risk of dementia and depression

- a 50% lower risk of colon cancer and type 2 diabetes

- a 35% lower risk of coronary heart disease and stroke.

The benefits of exercise are greater if one can raise the heart rate, breathe faster, and feel warmer. This degree of effort is called moderate-intensity activity. If the degree of the energy of your physical activity is harder, then this is known as vigorous-intensity activity. Researchers have shown that vigorous activity can bring more significant benefits than moderate activity.

A sedentary lifestyle is a modern problem.

Technology has made our lives more comfortable. We travel around by cars or get the public transport. Then, we spend hours and hours in front of a TV or computer screen. Nowadays, the majority of people have jobs that need little physical effort. Research indicates that many adults spend at least seven hours a day sitting down, on transport or in their leisure time. The most sedentary lifestyle is people over 65, as they spend at least ten hours each day sitting or lying down.

The United Kingdom Department of Health described inactivity as a silent killer. Evidence revealed again and again that sedentary behaviour is bad for our health. Bear in mind that it is important to increase our activity levels, and, at the same time, to decrease the amount of time we spend sitting down. A sedentary behaviour can carry terrible consequences like raising our risk of stroke, type 2 diabetes, and heart diseases, as well as obesity or weight gain.

It can be challenging nowadays to be more active or pro-active. Previous generations performed natural activities through work and manual labour, but today it is harder to find ways to keep us moving and integrate activity into our daily lives/habits.

## 8.3 - What habits should we adopt to help us exercise more?

Exercise has great attributes to help us refresh our body cells. It is an excellent antidote for depression and, in general, it makes you feel good about yourself.

Medical experts recommend adults try to accomplish at least 150 minutes of exercise every a week through a varies of activities.

The best way to get moving is to do exercises as a part of our daily life. You should make it a habit to walk or bicycle instead of driving a car. That's the way it works; the more you do, the easier it is to take part in activities (sports/exercises), and it will help you to achieve a healthier lifestyle.

There are tips on how to implement new habits to build and develop your physical activity on a daily basis. It seems there is an excuse for everything when we don't want to do exercise. I know some people who make all kind of reasons for not exercising. They keep saying they don't have the time. But, like anything else that's important, one has to prioritise and put it in their schedule. You can break your activity into 15-minute chunks. There are even apps that can help you to fit in a daily 15-minute walk.

Another common blocker that prevents you from getting more active is thinking you are too tired after a long day at work, and exercise might not be on the top of your list. The tiredness you may feel is mainly mental fatigue, and engaging in some exercise will benefit you, and you will feel more energised.

Another excuse is that you don't have the willpower. Maybe you would get motivated if you could exercise with a family member or a friend. Or, you could join a local club to help you get motivated.

If you do not want to join gyms or clubs, a simple way to keep you fit is running upstairs. It's a fantastic way to build muscle and improve your overall cardiovascular fitness. I had a friend that was addicted to keeping healthy and routinely did as many exercises as he could. For instance, he always encouraged me to take the stairs, instead of the lift. Thanks to him, I got into the habit of running up the stairs, rather than taking an escalator.

It was an excellent habit indeed, and this simple exercise helps you to elevate your heart rate so that more oxygenated blood is circulated throughout your body. A good and safe way of practising is keeping a faster pace going up the stairs and walking down normally. And, if you have the strength and coordination of doing this exercise and you can take two steps at a time, go for it. This will make sure that your muscles work harder and you will burn more calories. The more steps you can climb, the harder your body will work.

Don't get into the habit of saying that exercise is hard work, or that you have to go to the gym, or you have to subscribe to a club. Exercise, as you have just seen, can be available to anyone. Choose the activity you enjoy. Get into the habit and start slowly. Make small habits and build up gradually. By doing it this way, you will make progress, and you will enjoy it more.

To make the habit stick, it is very important to set a time for physical activity and stick to it. It is more probable that you will find the time to exercise if you do it at the same time every day.

By splitting your activities throughout the day, you can accomplish your target in bouts of ten minutes or more.

Create the habit to walk your children to and from school. By doing this, it also creates a good habit for your children and helps them develop a pattern of physical activity.

Be active with your child, because there are lots of good reasons to get moving. Research reveals that physical activity can help to improve social skills, self-confidence, and behaviour. Some other reasons are to develop coordination, develop attention levels and performance at school, maintain a healthy weight, sleep better, and improve your mood and feel good.

In general, exercise enhances your health not only physically but mentally as well. Some  activities that you could be involved are swimming, or playing in the garden or park. Go to work by walking or cycling. If work is too far, simply get off the bus or tube two or three stops before your destination. A good habit your children need to follow is your level of activity. It is more likely that if you are a physical active parent, then your children will be too, so lead by example.

Get into the habit of encouraging your child to do more exercise by himself/herself or with friends, such as riding their bikes or playing chase, instead of watching TV. Let the child be involved in picking which exercises or physical activity they like the most. Some kids like running around or dancing. Perhaps you can take the children out for a bike ride. That's a fun activity for the whole family. Strength and flexibility exercises are excellent for healthy bones, joint pains, and muscle strength.

Exercise is good and does wonders for your general wellbeing and mental health. It is also associated with a longer life, and it diminishes the risk of different diseases. Exercise is terrific for a healthier and a better lifestyle.

# Chapter 9:
# How to Lose Weight and Be Happy

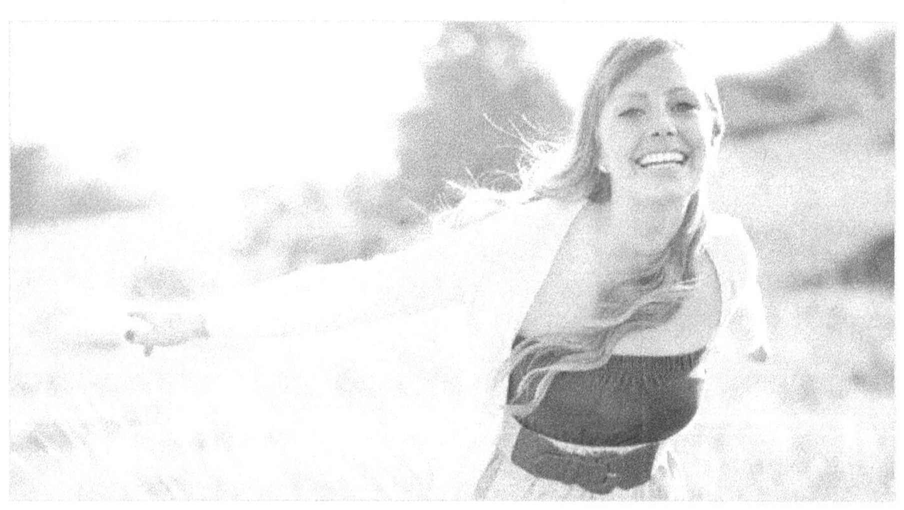

Being happy will prolong your life

# 9.1 - What is your ideal weight?

Obviously, when you are happy with yourself, you have a better self-image, and your intake of mood-boosting foods high in sugar and fat is unlikely if you are already happy.

Creating an environment for weight loss is essential. It is of consideration that our brain works in mysterious ways and produces neurochemistry that creates happiness. The most popular ways of boosting your serotonin levels are socialising with friends, by exercising, or by being outdoors in sunlight. Health practitioners revealed that this happiness seems potentially more responsible for weight loss, and it is similar to the number of calories you burn while you are in a gym.

Let me explain further. We will compare two events on how to lose weight. Let's imagine that you go to a gym to burn 600 calories in an hour. You despise it, but you are desperate to lose weight, so you go anyway. On the other hand, your friend is having the time of her life by spending her time with friends and meandering around the lake. They are breathless only because they share so much laughter. Laughing, in the end, loses similar or more weight than when you exercise. Yes, different factors may come into play, but studies have revealed that loving what you do is very beneficial for your health and your waistline.

The thing is that when you are happy, you are more likely to be committed to things you know you ought to do. Therefore, if you choose to exercise, make sure you choose the one you enjoy (whether or not it burns the most calories). Your state of happiness helps to improve your hormone balance and develop an environment conducive to weight loss.

Our mood is a tricky thing. For no reason, sometimes our mood can shift, changing our outlook on life completely. We can go from peaceful to angry, from happy to sad, and this can affect our perception of everything. Research has shown how attitudes and moods can influence work, relationships, and your general quality of life.

Depression and boredom are emotions known to trigger binge eating, which can cause weight gain. However, if you shift your attitude to a positive mood, it can affect your weight loss. For instance, if you start your day with a happy outlook, your mood keeps you going by having a satisfied feeling, and you are enthusiastic throughout the day. Being happy not only affects your attitude towards the people you love and your work, it also affects your weight loss. A confident individual sees the things that he or she has accomplished rather than focusing on what they have not achieved.

## 9.2 - What should I eat?

You may ask: how many calories should you eat a day to lose weight? But, then there are the good calories and the bad calories.

We are bombarded by social media to live a healthy lifestyle and make sure we do the right things, yet so many of us get it wrong. So, if your objective is to lose some weight, do not look any further. Here are some key factors you need to know to obtain the outcome you would like to have.

You need to remember that the average number of calories that you need will depends on your age, muscles mass, current weight, activity levels, and gender.

The amount of calories that one needs correlates directly with the activity levels of that person. For instance, on average, a small female doing less than an hour of exercise per day will need approximately 1400 to 1600 calories per day. On the other hand, a male will require roughly between 1800 to 2200 calories per day.

One of the methods that you can use to identify the level of your health concerning your body weight  is known as the body mass index (BMI). The BMI measures whether you are a healthy weight for your height. And this is calculated by dividing your weight in kilograms by the square of your height in metres.

For instance, my body mass index is 19.0. What I did was take my weight of 50 kg and divide it by my height in metres, which is 1.62 m , then divided the answer (which is 30.8) by my height again to get my BMI, which is 19.0.

For most adults, a BMI of 18.5 to 24.9 means you are a healthy weight. A BMI of 25 to 29.9 means you are overweight.

A BMI between 30 to 39.9 means you are obese, and above 40 means you are severely obese.

Another way to measure your excess fat is your waist circumference, which is a tool used as an additional measure in individuals who are overweight and moderately obese. Regardless of your height or BMI, you should lose weight if your waistline is: 94 cm (37 in) or more for men and women with a waist circumference of 80 cm (31.5 in) or more. The presence of abdominal fat goes hand in hand with disease risk, such as stroke, heart disease, or type 2 diabetes.

Health care practitioners used to think body fat was inert, but it is not. This fat is toxic, as fat tissues produce hormones and pro-inflammatory chemicals that regulate your metabolism, and that can lead to the progression of artery hardening, and the development of heart conditions or cancers. That is why it so important to keep your body weight down, and be aware of it and be willing to do something about it. You can get many biological benefits by losing weight and then you will feel amazing.

As an individual who is overweight, the initial goal of losing weight is to reduce your body weight by about ten percent. This takes approximately six months, depending on how much weight one has to lose. One can safely lose weight from one to three pounds per week. If you are into the obese group, health professionals recommend you undergo weight loss treatment.

If your BMI reveals that you are overweight, it is ideal for you to lose weight. It is important to consider that a weight loss treatment is fundamental and recommended, especially if you have more than two risk factors. These risk factors can include individuals who are inactive or people who smoke.

Let me introduce my friend, Olga. Olga had a weight problem. She was not pleased with her weight and health status, but overall, she was happy with herself and happy about the achievements she had reached in life. Being happy made it easy for her to stay on track in losing weight. Thus, her happy mood helped her to stay focused and committed to healthy habits, and they contributed to her 25-pound weight loss over one year.

Now, meet Victor. He used to be my neighbour. He was a very overwhelmed individual consumed with stress over changes in his life. Even though he had to lose less weight than Olga, he remained focused on the challenges and problems rather than on the opportunities. He chose something that he was not committed to doing for his body, due to his workaholic tendencies, and he usually stuck with his junk food and fizzy drinks habits.

These comparison cases can be a reflection of many of us. Now, if you are Olga, lucky you! Make sure that you feed that happiness on a regular basis by expressing gratitude, a balanced diet, and a selection of exercises that you enjoy the most to do.

If instead, you are like Victor, please do not despair. You are not alone. Be aware if you have a little of the half-empty attitude at first.

For many years, and I should say decades, people have been trying to lose weight in different ways, mainly by undertaking diets that did not work. These diets may give you the illusion of losing, but after a while, you gain your weight back. Our body is like an elastic band: if you push it too much, it can break.

Each of us is unique. No! No! No! It is not a cliché. It is a fact. It is just the way our brain works and how our metabolism function is unique.

Be mindful that when you do something, do it in a way that will benefit *you*. Do not follow others or the masses.

For years, the food industries and health professionals told us that losing weight and maintaining that loss was exclusively about calories consumed and calories burned. That way of losing weight was demonstrated as being a complete fiasco.

The concept that all calories are perceived as equal is not true. Think about it. You can see that healthy foods like fruits or vegetables don't have the same level of calories as junk food. So, considering only how many calories each food item contains is very misleading indeed.

Nutritionists disagree with the calories in / calories out approach to dieting. They reported that maintaining a healthy lifestyle is very important with weight loss. Just because someone has lost weight, doesn't necessarily mean he or she is healthy. Some people can reach the stage where losing weight is everything. It is vital to eat things of nutritional value to maintain your body's health on the CICO (Calories In, Calories Out) diet. Thus, for instance, you could eat candy bars or crisps exclusively for your daily calorie allotment and still lose weight, but you would eventually suffer from malnutrition.

Also, nutritional experts manifest that pursuing fad diets that are unsustainable in the long term (they avoid or heavily restrict the main key food groups: proteins, carbohydrates, and fats) may lead to severe long-term diseases, such as a higher risk for obesity and heart conditions.

Unfortunately, there are many misleading messages out there, about diets, which foods to eat, and nutrition. The food industry and the way they sell their products is very much based on a clever use of marketing and buzz words on food and drink products, which make us believe some food products are healthy when, in reality, they are not.

Food companies have a tendency of marketing products as healthy, even though they might not be a healthier option in all aspects. For instance, you may wish to eat a product that has fruit and looks healthy, but in fact, it may not contain much fruit at all.

Some tips to identify whether a product is healthy or not is easy.

Usually, food products that come in a packet are often not as healthy as raw, non- processed foods, particularly when it comes to fruits and vegetables. Therefore, buying hardly prepared food products is best.

If you buy prepared foods in packets, get into the proper habit of checking the back of the pack for the nutrition label and ingredients. On the label, the main thing you need to check for is the ingredients list. If there is a long list of ingredients, it is a very processed product and, more than likely, it is not that good for you.

Things to look at in the nutritional information on the product label are saturated fats, sugars (carbohydrates), and salt. By doing this, you will have a better idea of the product in question, and you can compare two products and choose the one with the better ingredients.

A guide to help you to understand sugar (carbohydrate), fat, and salt contents in product labels, in 100 grams, aim for the following:

- Sugar- approximately 5 g for food, and less than 2.5 g for drinks

- Total fat approximately 3 g for food, and less than 1.5 g for drinks

- Saturated fat, approximately 1.5 g for food, and less than 0.75 g for drinks

- Sodium (salt), approximately 120 mgs for food, and less than 120 mgs for drinks.

Get into the habit of eating fruit rather than drinking juice. Juice is not as good an option as fruit. Either way, one is better off to have a piece of fruit for the high levels of fibre and a glass of water.

Another consideration is the gluten-free biscuits; the fact that they are gluten-free does not automatically make them healthy. Bear in mind, that they are higher in fat and sugar, as they have to replace the taste and texture. Only for those who suffer from a coeliac condition or are diagnosed with a gluten intolerance should eat them as a healthy option, but in moderation.

Indulging once in a while makes it easier to eat well the rest of the time. Moreover, you are not alone. If you need somebody to help you with your daily life habits, there are smart, accessible, and engaging, foodists who can help you to set up your eating habits. They will help you match your lifestyle and your food preferences, making sure the path you choose works for you in the short- and long-term. Not only will you permanently build happier and healthier food habits into your daily life, but you'll also lose weight and enjoy food like never before. Embrace that burning desire to make the most of your life! Start with looking after your body, as you have never done it before, and start feeling amazing.

## 9.3 - What habits should you implement to help you lose weight?

Drink water - always remember to drink plenty of water to keep your energy levels high, and drink a glass of water before your meals to help you to lose weight.

Get grounded - meditation, particularly walks on green grass (it is known as forest bathing), which can lead to a sensation of peace and calm in your inner self.

Practices like meditation help you to reduce stress and to regain a centred feeling, and it will help you recover that happiness element that, in turn, will make you take better care of yourself. Being mindful of yourself and your surroundings in the present moment is a great habit, so make it part of your life too.

Stretching exercises are a good habit to maintain and get oxygen delivered to all your extremities and add in a few more deep breaths now and then.

Get a hug - yep, there is a cuddle hormone called oxytocin, which is another feel-good catalyst. A simple hug with another person, or even a pet, helps to decrease your anxiety and increase your happiness.

Employees of a large firm researched healthy people's habits. Among them are physical activity, forgiveness, food portion size, adequate sleep, trying something new, strength and flexibility, laughter, family and friends, addressing addictive behaviours, a calm mind, and gratitude.

Next, I will explain some of those healthy habits that contribute to a healthy and happy lifestyle, which, in the long run, is to lose weight.

Physical activity: let's make exercise a fun thing to do, rather than being a penance. For instance, you should consider getting a portable stepping or pedalling device that fits at your workstation. Another good habit is to include at least a ten-minute walk during your lunchtime.

You should also consider taking breaks from sitting. Get into the habit of stretching yourself or walking for a few minutes every hour while you're at work or relaxing at home.

Forgiveness – nowadays, we live a time of lawsuits, and sometimes mercy is only a concept from biblical times.

But, research suggests that forgiveness can have many health benefits. One health benefit is the ability to minimise the adverse effects (feelings of anger, depression, or tension). The reduction of these emotions can have beneficial effects, such as decreasing your blood pressure, and it could have immune system benefits. Thus, the lack of forgiveness can lead to health consequences like increased levels of negative emotion, and that would affect your health.

So, forgiving unconditionally could mean a longer lifespan. Forgiveness is cultivatable and can be developed through several methods, including practising empathy or adequately expressing your feelings.

Go for new changes of your daily foods to activate your passion for food. Explore a local farmers market, or take up gardening. These are fun ways be more active and explore new foods, new tastes, and new flavours.

Adequate sleep - studies revealed that the lack of sleep has a link to health problems, such as diabetes, obesity, and heart conditions. Yes, a good quality sleep makes you feel better and happier. Thus, adequate sleep is a crucial factor for a healthy life, as it has health benefits on your heart, mind, and weight. If you sleep better, you feel and live better. It's pretty clear. And I'm not going to say how much you need to sleep. Every individual requires more or less time of sleeping than another. Go with your body clock to see how much sleep is adequate for you. If, when you wake up in the morning, you feel fresh and energetic, that means you've had a good rest.

Try something new every day - we live a fast life, and its' easy to create a comfortable routine. Before you know it, you're talking the same topics with your workmates, taking the same route to work, and doing the same mundane and unfulfilling tasks every day. Trying something new is essential to incorporate brain stimulation. You should try a new social engagement like learning tai chi, dancing, or playing a sport. Studies revealed that physical activities contribute to the release of cellular growth factors that are vital for neurogenesis (the growth of new cells), which, at the same time, leads to a healthier and longer life.

Laughter is a great habit that you need in your daily life, and it can actually improve your health. Laughter is the best method to make you feel happy.  Laughter is the best medicine, it strengthens your immune system, minimises pain, and acts as a protector from the damaging effects of stress. By seeking out more opportunities for humour and laughter, though, you can improve your emotional health, strengthen your relationships, find greater happiness, and even add years to your life. Laughter triggers the release of endorphins, the body's natural feel-good chemicals. Endorphins promote an overall sense of well-being, and they can even temporarily relieve pain.

A good tip for when you are bored - instead of snacking, try an exercise video, dance, or go for a walk. Walks can be more enjoyable when you have a dog, and your dog will never let you forget to go for a walk. It will unconsciously become part of you, and not something compulsory that you have to do.

Make your leisure time active time, like going bowling, playing active games, or enrolling in fitness classes at local parks, gyms, or schools.

Your inner engineering is inclusive of your inner strengths of love, contentment, and peacefulness, as well confidence, resilience, and determination. These strengths help you to face the daily things in life, such as recovering from stress, getting things done at home or work, keeping up with your well-being, and being patient and caring towards others. The inner strengths are developed throughout time. Thus, it is essential as a reminder that these strengths grow through positive experiences. Therefore, we need to focus on decreasing on what is negative and increase what is positive.

# Chapter 10:
# Health

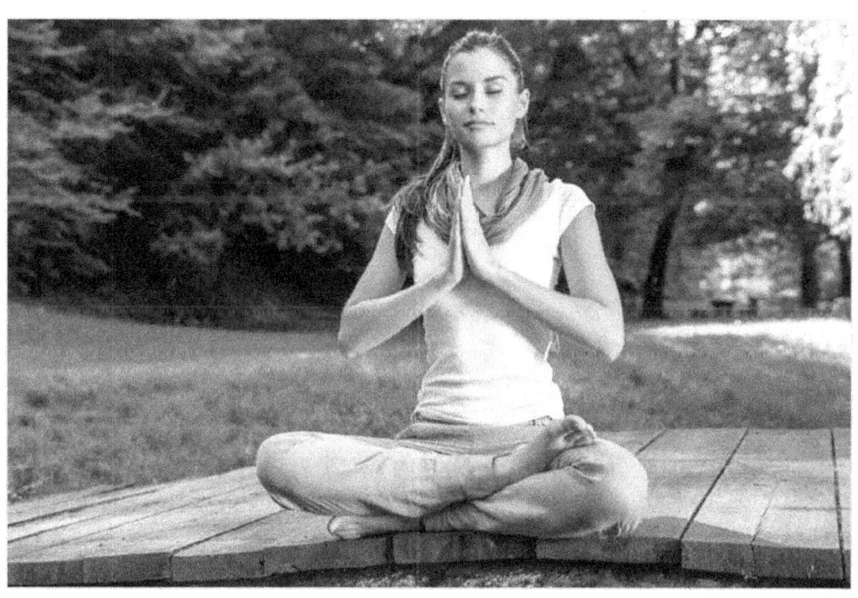

Meditation will help you to become healthier

## 10.1 - What is health?

One of the definitions of *health* by the World Health Organisation in 1948 is:

Health is a state of complete physical, mental, and social well-being and not merely the absence of disease or infirmity.

However, health can also be defined as the ability to adapt to one's environment. It is not a fixed entity, and it differs for every individual according to his/her circumstances. Health is described not by the doctor, but by the person, depending on the individual's functional needs.

Good health is primordial to tackle any stress and to help you live a long and active life. Let's take it as an inspiration and not moan about everything. Life is what it is, and groaning about it will lead us nowhere. LIFE is a gift, and you should always, always try to make the most of it!

There are different types of health. By this, I mean physical, spiritual, and mental health.

You are considered to have a good physical health when you experience that your bodily functions are working at peak performance. It's not just a lack of illness, but the performance of regular exercise, proper nutrition, and appropriate rest.

Being healthy physically helps you to minimise the risk of a disease or injury. Also, for you to achieve good health, it is essential to keep up with a good standard of health criteria, such as proper hygiene and avoiding the use of tobacco, alcohol, or recreational drugs.

On the other hand, mental health is associated with your psychological, social, and emotional wellbeing. Thus, mental health is as important as physical health to a full, active lifestyle.

Mental health is about not only not being depressed or anxious, or being free of any disorders, it also depends on your ability to feel safe and secure, enjoy life, achieve balance, adapt to adversity, and accomplish your full potential. Thus, mental and physical health are connected. If chronic diseases affect an individual's ability to fulfil their regular tasks, this may lead to stress and depression, due to financial problems. Another illustration of the physical and mental connection in our body is a mental illness like anorexia nervosa, which can affect body weight and function. So, it is vital to approach health as a whole, rather than its different types.

The main factors that can have an impact on our health are genetics, our environment, relationships with friends and family, education level, and income. Thus, the social and economic environment involves how wealthy a family or community is. The physical environment involves the pollution levels of that community. And the individual's characteristics and behaviours are affected by the genes that an individual is born with and their lifestyle choices.

Statistics have shown that the highest socioeconomic class has an increased chance to enjoy good health, a good education, a better well-paid job, and they can afford an excellent healthcare facility.

On the other hand, people who have a lower socioeconomic status are more prone to experience stresses associated with daily living, like marital separation, unemployment, financial difficulties, discrimination, and marginalisation. All these factors contribute to the risk of poor health. Another consideration that can affect health is a cultural factor. The customs and traditions of your country or family's traditions can have a good or bad impact on your health.

For instance, Mediterranean communities tend to consume high amounts of vegetables, fruits, and olives, and they eat as a family, compared to other cultures with a high intake of junk food.

So, how you deal with stress will affect your health negatively or positively. Individuals who drink, smoke, or take drugs are likely to suffer from more health issues later than somebody who deals with stress through balanced nutrition and exercise. One of the benefits of doing exercise is to relieve stress and, therefore, lower cortisol levels. The cortisol hormone is associated with the stress hormone. Also, physical activity is excellent for releasing endorphins and improving your mood and your health as a whole.

As they say, prevention is better than a cure. So, the best way to keep up your health is to preserve it through a good lifestyle, rather than waiting until you get sick to put things right.

Therefore, to keep up our wellness and optimal health is a lifelong, daily commitment. There are vital steps that can help us to maximise our health. Some of these steps are nutritious eating patterns, sourced as naturally as possible; screening health conditions that may present a risk; regular exercising; engaging in activities that have a purpose and meaning to others; keeping a positive outlook; and having an appreciation of what you are and have.

## 10.2 - Some of the healthiest foods of all time that can make you very happy

Make it a habit to consume the following foods:

**Blackberries** are good for you due to a high level of vitamins K, C, manganese and fibre, which can give you a full and satisfied sensation after eating them. Also, studies revealed that blackberries are related to health benefits of the body and mind, such as minimising the rate of cognitive decline. The vibrant colour of the blackberries can also help to reduce inflammation and strengthen the immune system.

**Coconut** has healthy benefits. It contains a good helping of potassium, which can contribute to curbing a stroke risk. And, it can be eaten, for example, when you sprinkle it on a raw kale or collard green salad.

**Mango** is good for you thanks to its high percentage of antioxidants and vitamins, in particular vitamin A. A mango provides 45% of your daily Vitamin A requirement.

**Harissa** is a spicy chilli paste or powder, and it is a mixture of healthy ingredients like garlic, olive oil, chilli peppers, and spices. This food is healthy because of a compound it contains known as capsaicin, which is helpful for relieving pain and has cancer-protective effects.

**Goat cheese** has less fat per serving than most cheeses. It is good for you because it contains calcium, protein, and 3% of your iron needs in just one ounce. Moreover, researchers reported that compared to cow milk, goat milk maximises iron absorption and benefits your bones.

**Popcorn**: if you go for a snack go for popcorn, as it is good for you due to the high level of fibre. And, of course, we are not referring to movie / theatre popcorn. Make your popcorn on the stove without melted butter and salty seasonings. It is fast and straightforward.

**Grass-fed beef** has less saturated fat than conventional grain-fed beef, and it's higher in good fats like conjugated linoleic acid, monounsaturated fatty acids, and omega-3s. Furthermore, it is an excellent source of iron, and it is high in protein, which is essential for development and growth.

**Ghee** is right for you because it is clarified butter that is made by melting butter and skimming off some of the fat. It is used in Indian cuisines, and some people find it easier to digest. Its flavour is slightly nutty and can be used as an alternative to cooking oils or butter.

**Canned salmon** can be an alternative to fresh salmon; it is less expensive. It is good for you thanks to the excellent sources of vitamin D, which is good for calcium absorption and bone health, and it contains omega-3 fatty acids.

**Spirulina** is a blue-green alga, and it is good for you due to high levels of vitamins, antioxidants, and nutrients that protect cells. It is also a good vegetarian source of protein. To eat it, add a teaspoon to your morning natural smoothie or oatmeal.

**Lemon** is good for you, as it has high levels of vitamin C. This vitamin also contributes to protecting your cells from damage, and it is needed by the body to make collagen, which helps your wounds to heal.

**Tofu** is good for you, as it is a plant with a based protein source, and it is high in iron and calcium. Tofu also contains isoflavones, which help your heart health and reduce your risk of breast or prostate cancer. And it is delicious in salads.

**Dandelion greens**: these bitter greens are good for you since they are rich in vitamin C, B, potassium, iron, and calcium. All these vitamins are an ideal mix for healthy muscles and bones.

**Purple potatoes** are good for you for their richness in potassium, which is required for blood pressure management. What is different about these potatoes are their purple colour, which comes from anthocyanin, which is an antioxidant that helps your cardiovascular system stay healthy.

**Nutritional yeast** is good for you due to its complete protein with all nine relevant amino acids. It also possesses vitamin B, selenium, zinc, and fibre.

**Oysters** are good for you. This seafood contains a good source of omega 3s fatty acids, zinc, protein, calcium, iron, and vitamin B12. B12 is vital, as it contributes to the good health of your body's nerve and blood cells. Unfortunately, the data on their effectiveness as an aphrodisiac is less robust.

**Strawberries** are a great fruit for you, as they are a good source of vitamin C and other nutrients that contribute to keeping your metabolism and your bones healthy. Also, the research found that they have health properties that will lower your risk for a heart attack.

**Artichoke** is a vegetable with a meaty texture, and it is good for you as it is rich in vitamin C, K, folate, fibre, and plenty of antioxidants like anthocyanins and quercetin. When you buy an artichoke, make sure you buy one that is heavy and firm.

**Sauerkraut** is a fermented cabbage full of calcium, magnesium, copper, and sodium, and it is also high in protein. Like any other fermented foods, sauerkraut contains probiotics that benefit the gut and digestion.

**Spaghetti squash** is good for you for the highest content of water of all the winter squash. It contains a good source of calcium, vitamins A and C, and fibre.

**Apples** are good for you thanks to the type of fibre that helps to decrease cholesterol levels, leading to a heart-healthy snack, and they help to regulate digestion.

**Wild-caught cod** is a versatile fish, and it is available during the whole year. Cod is low in fat, but a high percentage of its fat is a good fat full of omega 3s fatty acids, which are good for you, as they help reduce cardiovascular disease risks.

**Rhubarb** is good for you thanks to its high content of vitamins and folate. A tip how to eat it: try pickling your rhubarb for a savoury kick.

**Purple cauliflower** is good for you thanks to the antioxidant known as anthocyanin. This vegetable is high in fibre; manganese; vitamins B6, K, and C; and folate. It is low in calories. All these compounds help with early brain development.

**Endive** is good for you as it contains fibre and inulin, which contributes to decreasing LDL cholesterol levels, which benefits the heart. It is a wonderful source of potassium, iron, beta-carotene, and vitamin B. It can be eaten raw or in salads or appetizers.

**Snap peas** are considered to be a healthy snack, as they full of nutrients (vitamins K, C, and A) and fibre, and they taste delicious when raw.

**Corn** is good for you, and it is the equivalent of one ear of corn to approximately the same high nutrients and calories as an apple. It also contains zeaxanthin and lutein, which are two phytochemicals that contribute to a healthy vision.

**Pumpkin** is not only for carving. It is a delicious food full of minerals like magnesium and potassium, and it is also rich in beta-carotene, which is good for the immune system. It has a high content of vitamin K (which is approximately 50% of your daily value), and it helps to prevent blood clotting.

**Kimchi** is the alternative Korean version of fermented cabbage, and it's good for you as its health benefits are similar to sauerkraut, which contains healthy probiotics that regulate digestion.

**Olives** are loaded with healthy fat that can help your brain and heart. Moreover, they are an important source of antioxidants that prevent the build-up of bad cholesterol in artery walls. They are also considered as being a fermented food, and thus have the health benefits of gut-friendly bacteria.

**Asparagus** is good for you thanks to a wealth of folate, which helps with different body functions, and they also have a high level of vitamins A, C, and K.

**Figs** are good for you for their high levels of vitamins A and C.

**Pork Tenderloin** is good for you, and this is a part of the pork that has been certified by the American Heart Association, indicating that it is heart-healthy meat. Also, it contains vitamin B, zinc, and it is high in protein.

**Kombucha** is good for you as it is a fermented drink full of probiotics, which optimize the healthy bacteria in your gut. It also helps with digestion and increases the absorption of nutrients from your food.

**Buckwheat** is a whole grain. It is good for you, it is rich in fibre, it is a complete protein, and it is gluten-free. It can be eaten in soups, or as the base for a dish instead of rice.

**Ginger root** is good for you as a remedy to help out with nausea and motion sickness. It is a very traditional remedy that has been used for thousands of years.

**Mint** is good for you as a natural remedy to treat digestive problems, and it is also considered to have anti-viral and antimicrobial effects.

**Carrots** are good for you, as they contain vitamin A, which helps your vision. Also, they are loaded with antioxidants like beta-carotene and lycopene. Lycopene is the same compound that gives tomatoes their bright red colour. Carrots may reduce risks of certain cancers.

**Ground sesame seeds**, known as tahini, are a good source of vitamin E, potassium, iron, and calcium. One tablespoon contains 110 mg of phosphorus, which is the essential nutrient for the formation of teeth and bones. Also, it contains vitamin B, which helps out with muscle contractions and a normal heartbeat.

**Basil** is the main ingredient in pesto. Extracts from basil leaves are loaded with antioxidant elements that fight inflammation. It is a versatile food thanks to its simple way to add a touch of nutrition to different recipes.

**Pistachios** are good for you because of their heart-healthy fats. They contain plenty of antioxidants, including, gamma-tocopherol, lutein, and beta-carotene. They also have a wealth of vitamin A, which is vital for vision and proper organ function.

**Spelt** is a grain, and it is becoming more and more popular. It is a good source of both soluble and insoluble fibre, thiamine, copper, niacin, vitamin B2, and magnesium. It has some health benefits in its fatty and amino acids, which are essential for all body functions. You can eat spelt with wild mushrooms soup with pasta.

**Sunflower seeds** are good for you, as they are high in vitamin E, which is an antioxidant that is good for your immune system. For instance, one ounce of sunflower seeds contains 7.4 mgs of vitamin E, which is approximately 37% of your daily value.

**Parsley** is good for you, as it is rich in many major vitamins that play a role in the immune system, bones, and the nervous system. It also contains flavonoids like luteolin or apigenin, which have some anti-inflammatory effects.

**Some of the unhealthiest foods that can make you very unhappy**

A junk drink like soda is considered one of the worse. This sugary drink is not your friend, it doesn't do any favours for your waistline, and it can erode your teeth. Also, it can affect your skin, anxiety levels, blood glucose, and hormones. Every time that you drink a fizzy drink, you receive no nutritional benefits whatsoever. In contrast, it contributes to increasing your glucose levels in your blood, as soda can contain up to eighteen teaspoons of refined sugar.

Also, soft drinks contain exuberant doses of artificial food dyes and preservatives like BVO (brominated vegetable oil). So, the next time you feel thirsty, do yourself a favour and take a glass of water with a splash of lime or lemon, or have 100% fruit juice.

Deli meats - nitrates may sound like a ticking time bomb, which in a certain form is not far from the truth, as deli meals are considered to have high levels of salt, additives, and preservatives. Among these products are salami, ham, or bologna. Over consumption of these products can increase your chances of cancer and heart disease.

If you need meat for sandwiches, get deli meats from a butcher. They contain fewer harmful preservatives than the packaged ones. A good tip is to buy a chicken breast and slice it into thin strips for sandwiches.

Artificial sweeteners - please be mindful that because artificial sweeteners (aspartame, neotame, saccharin, sucralose, etc.) contain fewer calories than refined white sugar, they are not healthy substitutes.

Bear in mind that if you need a touch of sweetness, you could try natural agave syrup or honey.

Margarine contains trans fats (or saturated or hydrogenated oils) that can lead to a heightened risk of strokes, heart disease, and bad cholesterol.

Get into the habit of skipping margarine and using mashed avocado or extra virgin olive oil for healthier options.

Bottled salad dressings - if you have a healthy and delicious meal, the worst thing you can do is drown your salad in bottled salad dressing. It will not make much difference if it is the fat-free or reduced-fat dressings, as they all contain high fructose corn syrup, sugar, and additives like caramel colouring. In the end, it's like pouring diet soda over your mixed greens.

For a healthier alternative to salad dressings, mix a few tablespoons of balsamic vinegar or apple cider vinegar with a bit of virgin olive oil.

Life is about moments with family sharing each other's company, having food together, eating, talking, and laughing.

Those precious moments are when we have happy times, and, yes, you want them to last as long as you can. Life is too short already. Don't make it shorter by eating the wrong stuff. Make it a habit and start today, to eat those foods that make you feel amazing.

## 10.3 - What habits should you implement to get and stay healthy?

Nowadays, everybody wants to look younger than their age, and a lot of people spend a significant amount of money to make themselves appear more youthful. It is said that the age one seems to be is based on far more than one's everyday habits. So, which habits should you avoid to look younger and healthier?

**Habit 1 – quit smoking**! Aaah! I know it's not a surprise, but, still, it seems that many need to be reminded. Give up smoking. Smoking is not suitable for our body as cigarettes and cigars contain chemicals that, once they are released into the air in the form of smoke, have a tendency to stain everything they come into contact with. And that includes eyes, teeth, hair, and even skin. Smoking can also badly damage the throat, lungs, and mouth. These damaging effects can alter one's voice, and they will sound much older than they are.

**Habit 2 - sleep enough hours**. Adults need roughly seven hours of sleep, and children need between eight and ten hours. The lack of sleeping can make us look and feel older than we are. Not being able to sleep enough robs us of the mental and physical energy we need to get through a typical day. A lack of sleep is hard on our bodies, like our primary and vital organs: the heart and the brain. The bottom line is that not sleeping the right number of hours and resting according to your body's needs, makes you look and feel years older.

**Habit 3 - avoid eating junk food**. The terrible habit of eating junk or fast food, from crisps to cookies or candies, is a vicious cycle. Let me explain. First, you eat fast food (which may taste good), but it leaves you feeling bloated, generally lousy, and tired. Then, because you feel bad with yourself for eating unforbidden food, you avoid doing the things that can help you to boost your energy and mood, such as go to the gym or playing sports.

Unfortunately, the cycle repeats, and once an individual gains weight, it can lead the person to no longer care about his/her appearance, and they struggle to eat stuff without fat, sugar, or grease. Unless one can break this habit, it's going to be very hard to get the idea of exercising regularly and eating healthy food, it becomes a foreign concept, and one can look older as a result.

**Habit 4 - exercise regularly**. One of the main keys to looking younger and being healthier is keeping in reasonable physical shape. The majority of people require a proper and balanced diet, full of fruits, vegetables, and lean proteins. But, another essential ingredient is to do physical activity on a daily basis. A good habit is to ensure that you exercise on a regular basis, and not randomly. Make sure you get in the habit of doing it, and once you do that, it will become automatic for you, and you will do it without realising it. The physical activity not only helps us to keep both our energy levels and our appearance but it also helps to boost our self-esteem.

**Habit 5 - take veggies seriously**. I know many people who just prefer to eat something else, rather than fruits or even vegetables. But try to introduce into your diet one piece of fruit on a daily or weekly basis, and get into the habit of eating a piece of fruit or a vegetable in your daily eating routine. The key here is to find vegetables that you enjoy eating. Remember they make you look younger and much healthier.

**Habit 6 - avoid binge drinking**. Alcohol can make us look older, because drinking alcohol—and especially drinking to excess—dehydrates our bodies and our skin. Dry skin is especially noticeable around your eyes, so they show the first signs of ageing. Even if you're in your twenties, preventative care now will keep your eyes looking healthy for years to come, instead of looking dry, sore, and rough.


Your health and appearance are positively influenced by increasing your emotional and mental well-being.

I have always been passionate about what I eat, and the importance of what we eat is paramount to how our eating habits can transform our lives for good or bad.

So, it is your choice. Which side do you want to be on?

We have a body that gives us everything that we need, and yet we take it for granted. We don't realise how fortunate we are. We are so concerned about the world and how chaotic it has become, but, really, who is our number one enemy? And for our body, I also mean our mind and spirit, which is the motor of our daily life and body.

A determined mind can do miracles with their body. If that determination is there and it is converted into good habits, the sky is our limit. We must believe in ourselves and decide what kind of body and mind we would like to have. Our body is the real weapon that we have, and we need to make things happen. You are the master of your destination, and this is my dedication to all those who reflect and identify with the belief that everything is possible when you change your bad habits to healthy habits and work as a whole towards feeling amazing.

# About the Author

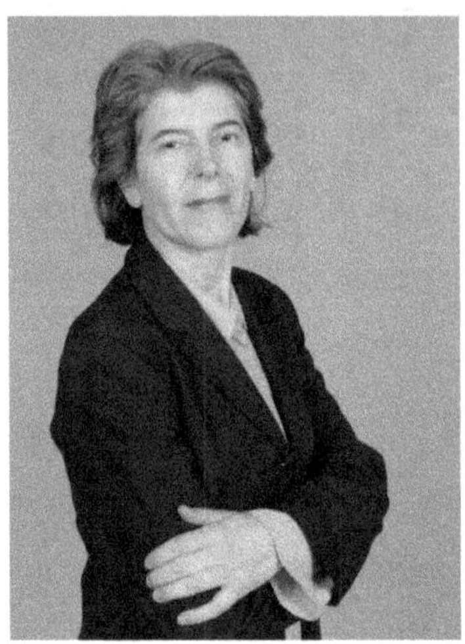

My dream is to make a difference in people's lives. In my case, it is to help children obtain clean, drinkable water and better sanitary conditions. By doing this, we could eradicate so many diseases, and, therefore, deaths. This is the basic right that any human being must have.

I would like to set up a project where a team of different professionals from all over the world volunteered their time. We would need architects, logistical engineers, mechanical engineers, educators, teachers, managers, and so on to build wells and set up more sustainable hygienic conditions where it is most needed.

That would be an amazing health habit for everyone. A project like this is what I mean to be a human being. We should be there for one another.

www.loallariz.com